JOHN MACLEAN was born in Sydney in 1966. A near-fatal accident in 1988 left him a paraplegic. He has since completed three Hawaii Ironman Triathlons, swum the English Channel, represented Australia at two Paralympic Games and completed the Sydney to Hobart Yacht Race. John lives in Sydney and today shares his lessons with a global audience (see www.johnmaclean.com.au). He also continues to help change the lives of children in wheelchairs through the John Maclean Foundation (www.jmf.com.au).

LYNNE COSSAR has worked as a journalist, writer and editor for Australian magazines and newspapers for 20 years. She has covered wars and famine in Africa, military coups in the Pacific and politics in South America and the United States. Her work has appeared in the *Good Weekend*, *The Age*, *Sunday Age*, *The Sydney Morning Herald*, *HQ Magazine* and *Business Review Weekly*. This is her first book. Lynne is married with two sports-loving sons, Max and Darcy, and lives in Bondi, Sydney.

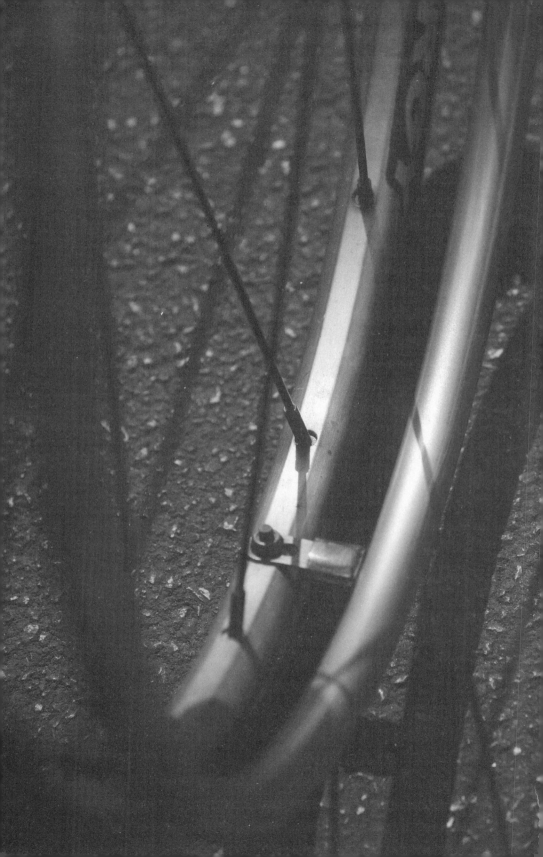

John
Maclean

full circle

One life, many lessons

with Lynne Cossar

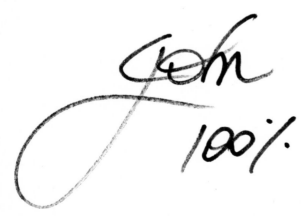

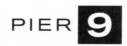

PIER 9

Published in 2009 by Pier 9, an imprint of Murdoch Books Pty Limited

Murdoch Books Australia
Pier 8/9
23 Hickson Road
Millers Point NSW 2000
Phone: +61 (0) 2 8220 2000
Fax: +61 (0) 2 8220 2558
www.murdochbooks.com.au

Murdoch Books UK Limited
Erico House, 6th Floor
93–99 Upper Richmond Road
Putney, London SW15 2TG
Phone: +44 (0) 20 8785 5995
Fax: +44 (0) 20 8785 5985
www.murdochbooks.co.uk

Writer: Lynne Cossar
Commissioning Editor: Colette Vella
Project Editor: Kate Fitzgerald
Copyeditor: Anne Savage
Design: Vivien Valk and Helen Beard

National Library of Australia Cataloguing-in-Publication Data
Author: Cossar, Lynne and Maclean, John, 1966–
Title: Full circle: one life many lessons/John Maclean; with Lynne Cossar.
ISBN: 9781741963977 (pbk.)
Subjects: Maclean, John, 1966–
               Athletes with disabilities--Australia--Biography.
               Achievement motivation.
               Competition (Psychology)
               Teamwork (Sports)
Other Authors/Contributors: Cossar, Lynne.
Dewey Number: 796.0456092

A catalogue record for this book is available from the British Library.

PRINTED IN AUSTRALIA.

FOREWORD

It is how we handle adversity that says much about the character and make-up of a person. In John Maclean I see a man who not only thrives on a challenge, but excels when the odds seem insurmountable. He is the guy you would want to be standing next to in the trenches doing battle; he is the player who you, the captain, rely on to kick the sideline conversion to win the grand final; the mentor that you want for your kids; the guy who makes a mockery of the 'dis' in disability.

After sustaining devastating injuries when struck by an eight-tonne truck as a promising twenty-two-year-old football player, John's life was abruptly turned upside down. It is impossible to comprehend one's mindset after such a traumatic event but here we are, some twenty years later, and John's achievements are simply astonishing.

He is driven, motivated and determined to continually meet, accept and conquer challenge after challenge, very often the first person to do so.

I was fortunate that our paths crossed when, during my

time as Australian of the Year (2004), I interviewed John for a high school teaching resource called *Chase your Dreams*. I was looking for role models to inspire the youth of Australia and believed John's story would motivate kids to make the most of what they had and to not waste their talents and opportunities. I was immediately impressed with John's incredible self belief and confidence that he could achieve anything he set his mind to, and also the fact that he was continually willing to put himself out of his comfort zone. To me this is how we fulfil our potential, and John's ability over the years to plot the seemingly impossible, then conquer it, provides us all with a stunning example that we are only limited by our imagination.

John Maclean is a winner, not just because of his achievements, but also because of the way in which he conducts himself and leads others. He has overcome family and personal tragedy, established his own charitable foundation, competed and excelled against able-bodied competitors, broken records, continually reinvented himself across various sports disciplines and, despite all of this, he remains a humble down-to-earth guy who always gives 100% and refuses to give in.

I, like many other Aussies, consider John to be a man of great integrity, and a role model we should all try to emulate.

All the best for the future, mate, and may you continue to challenge yourself and never be satisfied with the ordinary.

Steve Waugh AO

CONTENTS

Prologue—The Finish Line   1

Chapter One—Choosing to Live   5

Chapter Two—One Step at a Time   19

Chapter Three—Positive People   40

Chapter Four—Giving it 100 per cent   52

Chapter Five—Being Myself   66

Chapter Six—Setting Goals   72

Chapter Seven—Seeking the Truth   97

Chapter Eight—Persistence   103

Chapter Nine—Chasing my Dreams   126

Chapter Ten—See it, Believe it, Achieve it   149

Chapter Eleven—Finding Hope   174

Chapter Twelve—The Value of Balance   196

Chapter Thirteen—Humility   218

Chapter Fourteen—Never Giving Up   231

Chapter Fifteen—A Sense of Closure   258

Epilogue—A Future Bright with Promise   286

ACKNOWLEDGEMENTS

There are many people to acknowledge for this book, but most of all the people who saved my life all those years ago, those who looked after me at Westmead and Royal North Shore hospitals, and those who supported and guided me through recuperation and back into the game of life. My doctor, Atif Gabrael, and physiotherapist, Rob Standen, today keep 'my wheels on motion'.

I would also like to thank the members of my family and the friends, business colleagues and mentors who spent time revisiting my story with Lynne Cossar in order to put this book together.

John Young and David Knight deserve my utmost gratitude for their friendship and unwavering belief in me; Marc Robinson for providing balance and perspective over many years; Hans Hulsbosch, Ricky Jeffs, Ross Cochrane and Steve Nola for their ongoing support and direction; and Trent Taylor for his passion and belief in managing the John Maclean Foundation.

To the many supporters of the John Maclean Foundation and the members of the board—the work of the Foundation is enriched because of them.

To Gatorade, for their ongoing sponsorship and championship.

To Lynne Cossar, who transformed this book from a fledging idea to a fully formed reality, who put in tireless hours of research, investigation and writing to bring the story together.

To the team at Murdoch Books for a great experience and for producing book that I can be proud of. In particular, thanks to Juliet Rogers and Kay Scarlett for their commitment to me and to my story; Colette Vella and the editorial and design team for their direction, patience and sensitivity; and to the sales and marketing team for their enthusiasm and energy in ensuring my book has the best possible care as it finds its way to readers.

And, last but certainly not least, to my wife Amanda—for everything, but especially for giving my life new meaning.

John Maclean
Sydney, 2009

full circle

One life, many lessons

THE FINISH LINE

'Whether he wins a gold medal or not, he's done it again. He has qualified and he is racing for Australia and he is doing something else for the first time'
—DON MACLEAN, HALF-BROTHER

I knew it would soon be over. Sometimes time stands still, sometimes it races ahead so fast you can barely remember what transpired, sometimes it's important to hold onto the moment for as long as you can. I looked up at the afternoon sun and thought, 'This is it. This is what we have been waiting for and it's perfect. The sun is out. We've got a bit of a headwind.' It was a nice space to be in. Maybe it was the calm before the storm, but I was trying to take it all in—which I do on a regular basis before I finish a sporting event—because I knew I wouldn't be back. The job was almost done.

Now that the Beijing Paralympics have come and gone I won't row again. I have loved keeping fit through training. I have loved being on, and near, the water and in the open air, and enjoyed the camaraderie of the other rowers. I loved the opportunity for a gold medal. But do I love rowing? No. Love is not a word that comes to mind. I have left my boat and my oars to the Lakes Rowers Club, which operates out of the Sydney International Regatta Centre, which I hope will allow someone else to get into the sport. There was no yearning desire to continue. I wanted to move on in my life.

Australia is in lane 5, China in lane 3 and Brazil in lane 4, the lanes allocated to the three fastest heat finishers. The medals will be fought out between these three boats. An official calls out 'Australia!', and asks if we want to check for weed underneath the boat. Kathryn and I nod our heads. We are only minutes away from the start of the race of our lives.

I can't say I'm thinking wise thoughts at this critical moment. I'm a professional athlete, and as I wait for the siren and green light to signal the beginning of this final, my mind slips into autopilot. I know what I have to do. As a youngster I had trouble concentrating at school, but here, at the Shunyi Olympic Rowing-Canoeing Park in Beijing, China, there is nothing in the world that could possibly distract me.

We're away. Our first strokes are clean and efficient. I look straight ahead, focusing on my team-mate Kathryn and my own body. I feel the power surging through my arms and I know we are moving quickly through the water. Brazil skips to the front. This pair is explosive from the blocks and takes an early lead, just as we knew they would. At the 250-metre mark the time splits flash on the electronic scoreboard at the side of the course and the crowd erupts. Brazil is out in front. Their split is an extraordinarily fast 1:00.54. We are clear in second place, only 2.21 seconds behind, but China is breathing down our necks only another 0.79 seconds away in third. Just a boat length separates the three of us. It's going to be close. Our split is 1:02.75, almost exactly where we want to be. Our start is good—not perfect, but good. We've put ourselves in a position to win this race. Our plan is playing out, but all I can see is the shape of Kathryn's back as we try desperately to hit the rhythm that will take us to the finish line.

At 500 metres, Brazil is still in front, but now China is in second place, and we've dropped back slightly to third. Brazil's 500-metre split is 2:05.65, which means they've covered the second 250 metres in 1:05.11. They're slowing down a little—can they hold on? China is 2.54 seconds from the lead and gaining. We are 0.17 seconds behind China. Now less than a boat length separates the three of us.

Kathryn calls 'Now!', the signal that means I need to hold full power until the finish. It's not like I can find another gear—I'm already at full stretch. My heart rate is going through the roof and it's all I can do to hold it together. People are screaming in the grandstands on both sides of the course and I can see the other boats dropping off the pace—Italy, Great Britain and Poland are out of contention.

At the 750-metre mark, the lead changes again. China hits the front with a split of 3:14.39. We're in second place, only 0.66 seconds behind them and 0.53 seconds in front of Brazil. Brazil's going backwards after that scorching first 250 metres. It's a two-boat race now. Can we make up the difference? Can we hold our stroke and find something extra to rein in the Chinese rowers?

I know it's tight. I'm pulling, pulling, pulling. I'm not praying, I'm not thinking, just concentrating on making every stroke as long and hard and powerful as I can. Australia, China, Australia, China.

Next thing I know is the beep that signals the finish line ...

CHAPTER ONE

CHOOSING TO LIVE

*'As you can imagine he was totally devastated.
Here was a young man with a wonderful life
ahead of him in his twenties and suddenly it was
all gone'*
—ALEX MACLEAN, FATHER

I don't often park my car on the side of the road to think about life and the hand it's dealt me. But there is a particular spot on the M4 motorway, about 50 kilometres west of Sydney, where an unlikely confluence of events more than twenty years ago changed my life forever. And today that's where I find myself, sitting in the driver's seat of my red Holden station wagon looking for the first time at a dented, rusting guardrail, where for a period of time on 27 June 1988 I hovered between life and death.

The day had started promisingly. It was a Monday, one of those beautiful sunny days that Sydney delivers in winter—a special gift from nature. There wasn't a cloud in the sky, not a breath of wind in the air. I was twenty-two years old and, yes, a cocky young lad whose dream was to play first-grade rugby league football. I was playing for the Warragamba Wombats at the time. Warragamba is part country town, part regional centre, and country guys just love a nickname. Mine was 'Hollywood'. My best friend John Young, whom I met at Warragamba, says it was my long blond hair that was out of place with the football scene there. 'You had talent to burn, the six-pack, the hair and the attitude,' he explained to me once. 'But as the months went by they knew you didn't only look good, you could play, mate. Even now, everyone asks about you.'

I was fast. Sometimes I felt like I was running on air. Athletics was always my thing growing up in Tregear, a suburb in Sydney's west built in the post-war period when money was scarce and families struggled financially to raise their children. Even now the locals call it Fibro Central. It was a Housing Commission area, and although some people in our street, including my parents, went on to buy their homes from the Government, for others it wasn't an option. I wasn't much good at school, but I loved sport. It gave me a chance to excel. Now I am older, I suspect I competed as much for the love and attention it got me as for the medals and best and fairest awards.

Running set me apart from the pack, and I loved football training, but I wasn't much into sitting around the Warragamba clubrooms drinking beer with the boys after a training session. I wasn't a beer drinker and I was always keen to skip off and spend time with my girlfriend Michelle. Sunday nights were special, because occasionally we'd have my parents' house to ourselves for the evening.

Three weeks before that fateful day on the M4 I'd moved out of home into a rented three-bedroom, red brick house with my friend Michael Winter at Faulconbridge, a small town in the Blue Mountains, 78 kilometres west of Sydney. The Blue Mountains are so named because of the blue tinge they take on when viewed from a distance. I loved this part of the world, and later on its breathtaking natural beauty helped sustain me through my darkest days. Michael had been living away from home for a while—he was more independent than I was. Vacuuming and household tasks were not my forte, but Michael was very much into that sort of thing. I wouldn't have thought it, but I encouraged him to do what he enjoyed, all the while appreciating that it was to my advantage to be living with someone so well house-trained.

Leaving the nest for the first time is a sweet feeling. Life and its endless possibilities were opening up for me, and it was exciting—I was master of my own destiny, I could do what I wanted, when I wanted. The world was at my feet and I was ready to take it on. Giddy-up baby!

I'd been looking forward to that Monday. I had a rostered day off from my job as general assistant at Bennett Road Primary School in St Clair, about 37 kilometres from my new digs. I had the day mapped out. I was cross-training for a triathlon—my third—and had arranged to meet a mate in St Clair (near where I worked) who was constructing a tandem bike I intended to ride down the Blue Mountains with another mate, Colin Thomas. Our aim was to crack 100 kilometres an hour. Not rocket science, I admit, but we loved speed and had no fear.

I woke early, fixed myself a high-energy breakfast and put on my cycling gear. My new silver Malvern Star racing bike, worth $800 and purchased from the St Mary's bike shop, was my pride and joy. I was going to get out the front door, get on that Malvern Star and rip into it. Listening to a tape from a hip new band called Talking Heads on my Walkman, I headed off from Faulconbridge without a care in the world. The ride was exhilarating. I was an experienced cyclist, careful to stay left of the white line so as not to obstruct traffic, but keen to push as hard and fast as I could. At times I hit 80 kilometres an hour as the road began its descent into the Penrith valley, and I remember thinking, 'How good is this!' I'm not sure if I was laughing, but I know I was loving life as I hurtled down the hill.

I chose to live, not die.

I had a sandwich with the mate who was working on my tandem bike, then jumped back on the Malvern Star, eager to begin the journey home. It was about 12.30 in the afternoon. Travelling east in this part of the world is a whole lot easier than travelling west, but I looked forward to the physical challenge awaiting me as I tackled the hills on the way home. I liked the blood pumping through my veins and my heart racing at a ridiculous speed. I liked the endorphin rush and pushing myself to the limit.

I said goodbye and put on my helmet. And that's about where my memory of that sunny winter day ends. I know I made my way onto Mamre Road and onto the M4, which at that time was called the F4 and was a two-lane freeway each way, running east to west through western Sydney. The M4 is a notoriously dangerous road that links Sydney to the west of New South Wales, via a winding endurance-testing climb carved through the Blue Mountains followed by a sharp, spectacular descent to the grazing lands beyond. This motorway carries an extraordinary volume of traffic, much of it heavy-load trucks that travel at the maximum speed allowed, ferrying all sorts of cargo, their drivers facing strict deadline pressures and frequent traffic snarls.

I'm not a statistician, but even I know long odds when I see them. What would happen next was a million-to-one shot. If I had hesitated at any stage during the morning, if I had made one other stop to buy a bottle of water or Gatorade or go to the bathroom or to adjust the seat position on the bike, my life would have turned out differently. But I didn't. There was nothing—no warning, no premonition, no sudden chill or tingling up my spine—to suggest I should stop what I was doing, that danger lay ahead. I took the Mamre Road entrance ramp to the M4 and started pumping my legs to the driving beat of Talking Heads. I wouldn't have been thinking of much except the climb ahead and perhaps, if I was lucky, a sausage and mash dinner.

What brings two people together at a particular point in time, when they have no business or common ground to connect them in the first place? What forces are at work to entwine two people so intricately—so delicately—that their futures, to some degree, are linked by a shared past? Is it chance, a simple, uncomplicated coincidence? Is it a matter of statistics, simply being in the wrong place at the wrong time? Or is it something more? Are some things in life meant to be?

At the same time as I was powering into the bend on the on-ramp, a young truck driver, younger than me, was well into his shift. He had picked up his rig, an '85 Mitsubishi eight-tonne pantech, at the company depot in Parramatta, and was heading westbound on the M4 with a cargo of empty fire extinguishers. He was taking them to a company in Penrith that was going to powder-coat them before he delivered them to Brookvale and returned to Parramatta, where his work day would have ended around 5 pm. He usually moved furniture, but not this day.

I have no recollection—no blinding flash or deeply engrained subconscious image—of the time of impact. This is a blessing. I have never wanted the accident impregnated into my memory. What sort of recurring nightmare would that cause? I do know it took only an instant to change the course of my life. The truck hit me from behind. The full-on impact broke its left-hand indicator light and smashed the left headlight. It also caused a noise inside the cabin. In his record of interview, the truck driver said he was travelling west along the M4 and, while approaching the rear of a truck in front of him, started to merge into the right-hand lane to overtake it. He heard a slight bang and looked into the left-hand rear-vision mirror to see if he had collided with anything but, seeing nothing 'untoward', simply kept driving. After he'd overtaken and moved back into the left lane, he saw a motorcyclist beside him, frantically waving him down. He stopped, to be told he'd hit a cyclist. That cyclist was me.

A young teenager called Michael McKenzie, sitting in the back seat of his mother's car, witnessed the accident as they drove past in the opposite direction. He yelled at her to stop as he saw me flying through the air. Jumping out of the car, he dodged traffic on both sides of the freeway to reach me, certain I had to be dead. That mercy dash would have taken only a minute, but he still got to me after a priest, who must have been driving close behind the truck, and was already administering the last rites.

Calls to police and ambulance were made quickly, by whom I have no idea. One of the policemen first on the scene—who kept in touch with me periodically for years afterwards—says he remembers it like it was yesterday. Stationed at St Mary's, he was on patrol when the call came through. When he got to me the ambulance officers were already there. My body, he says, was 'twisted into a position that resembled a lifeless rag doll'. I was motionless. There was no visible blood, but not a lot of confidence among the people administering first aid. The policeman softly asked one of the ambulance officers whether I'd make it. The response was solemn: 'It's touch and go.'

The policeman, who asked not to be identified for the purposes of this book and who has since left the force, says he remembers seeing my beloved Malvern Star lying flattened and bowed on the side of the road. 'If that were the impact on the bike, which was made of aluminium, I thought at the time what the impact on your body must have been.' He recalls the truck driver's reaction: 'He was very upset and, I suspect, a little defensive. He didn't know what the consequences of his action would be.' The truck driver was later charged with negligent driving. He admitted to taking his eyes off the rear-vision mirror as he checked the road ahead to change lanes and overtake.

One thought stayed with the policeman for years: 'It was just such a perfect day. I empathised with you being out there cycling on such a beautiful afternoon.'

My injuries were massive. Westmead Hospital, which is 25 kilometres from where the accident occurred, and where I was rushed by ambulance, listed them in typical medical jargon: bacterial pneumonia, pulmonary contusion, retroperitoneal haemorrhage, head trauma, chest trauma, vertebral trauma, pelvic trauma, extremity fractures, vertebral fracture, pelvic fracture and other fractures.

In short, I had broken my back in three places, my pelvis in four places and my right arm in two places. I had fractured ribs on the left side of my body, a fractured sternum and a closed head injury, both lungs were punctured, and the ligament behind my right knee was ripped from its moorings. And I won't even talk about the gravel rash—yet. Bike gear doesn't offer much protection against gravel rash. In shock and mercifully unconscious, I was given seven units of blood when I arrived in the Intensive Care Unit. My condition was listed as critical.

The first time the word 'paraplegia' entered my world was that day. It was not said out loud—nor would I have been aware of it if it was—but it was one of the first words noted in my medical records when it became clear after a CT scan that the accident had damaged my spinal cord. The word flew off the page at me the first time I read it recently, but more chilling were the diagrams of my body, indicating where there was movement and feeling and where there was not. It was noted early that I needed a spinal bed if possible—and that the chaplain had been called to be with my parents.

It was my mother Anne who took the call from Westmead Hospital that alerted the family to my accident. She was told they thought I had a broken pelvis. Mum remembers no urgency in the voice on the other end of the phone, nor getting any sense that the accident was more serious than that. She rang Dad, who was at his cleaning job at Penrith Police Station. Together they drove to Westmead, explained who they were at reception, and were taken to a room where they sat by themselves for a very long time. Mum says they were getting concerned even before the hospital chaplain walked in and asked, 'Have you seen anyone yet?' When someone says that in a hospital you don't have to be Einstein to know that something is terribly wrong.

I think my parents were in shock. My dad, Alex, was the one who had the conversation with the ICU doctor about the seriousness of my injuries. The doctor didn't think I would survive the night, telling him, 'Your son's injuries are massive, just incredible.' When they were taken through to ICU to see me, Mum remembers I was swathed in bandages. She believes to this day that if I hadn't been so fit I wouldn't have survived.

Not one member of my family who saw me in the first few days after the accident can yet talk about it without crying. I had gone from being a cocky, outgoing, physical young man to someone they barely recognised. One minute I was full of life; the next I was fighting for it. That sudden transition is now, even twenty years later, a memory they find hard to process. Except, perhaps, my dad, who had worked for years as a policeman in Glasgow, pulling dead bodies out of lakes and knocking on doors in the middle of the night to tell people their loved ones had been killed or injured. There is a stoicism about his generation of males, and I believe my dad is more inured than most to life's tragedies because he has seen so many of them. That's not to say my accident didn't rock him to the core. Not long after he and Mum got to Westmead, he was asked to sign consent forms for an operation I needed urgently to fix my broken arm. His signatures on those forms are the shakiest I have ever seen him pen. As time went on, I would cry on his shoulder more than once about my plight and confide in him my fears about the future. More than once he cried too.

I have said already I have no memory of this sequence of events. But I do know that at some critical point after the accident, I chose to live, not die. It wasn't a tick-a-box, choose life not death scenario. There were no white lights or angels or doors opening with a willowy figure beckoning me forward. It was subtler than that. I sensed I could move in one of two directions: I could choose to close my eyes and sink my head into a soft pillow on a comfy bed and rest my tired and broken body. Or I could hold on. I could fight. I could live. There was no real choice for me—I wasn't done with life just yet.

Now, sitting in my Holden on the side of the M4, only 10 metres from where I was hit by that truck, I am not sure whether that near-death experience happened right here, or in the ambulance that rushed me to Westmead with sirens blaring. Maybe it happened in the ICU, where a team of highly skilled doctors and nurses were the ones who saved my life, and to whom I am eternally grateful. If I were pushed to pick one of those three places, I would say it was probably here, on the M4.

I have driven past this guardrail many times since the accident. I had even stopped there twice before: once with John Young, when we were training together for a triathlon, and once when I was hand-cycling from Brisbane to Melbourne to raise money for the foundation I set up to help kids in wheelchairs. I admit to having felt a tingle up the spine on both those occasions. Some people take this the wrong way. It wasn't a haunted feeling. It was more a sense of: 'I'm here, I'm back.' I guess it's like when you're a little kid and you fall off your bike and your mum or dad tells you to get back on and keep going. I'm still here. I'm back on a bike. It happens to be a hand-cycle rather than a conventional pushbike, but I'm still doing what I love to do. So I guess that's what I mean by a sense of being back. I'm back in the game of life.

I can't change what occurred twenty years ago, but I have tried not to let it change who I am or what I love to do—and that's sport.

This time, however, I have brought with me the photographs of the accident taken by the police forensic squad. I have looked at these photographs before, but not in this context. Not while sitting in my car, with the trucks thundering past at 110 kilometres an hour making it shake, reminding me so starkly of the force of the impact my body sustained all those years ago. There is a photograph that shows me lying on the road shoulder, with people who look like ambulance officers working over me. It's an awful photograph, not least because there are four people standing about 20 metres away. They say a picture is worth a thousand words and in this case it's true. These people look shocked and uncertain. It's the look I imagine you get when you are watching a disaster unfold before you and you don't know whether the victim is going to live or die, or perhaps already has passed away. There is another photograph of the truck that hit me. Its number plate has been rather amateurishly painted over with correction fluid, but you can see the damaged left headlight and broken indicator light.

I came here with these photographs as part of a road trip through my life. One of the aims of the journey was to jog my memory for the purposes of this book. But I also needed to close the page on this chapter of my life so I could begin the next one.

One of my favourite movies is the Academy-Award-winning film *Forrest Gump*, whose main character of the same name is played by Tom Hanks. Born with a twisted spine and less than stellar brain power, Forrest goes on to achieve amazing feats in his life, supported all the way by his mother. Throughout the film, Forrest likes to quote his mother. One of her truisms stuck with me. 'My Mama always said you've got to put the past behind you before you can move on,' Forrest said. It was time I did that, too.

Though I'd looked at these photographs before, now I felt as if I were seeing them for the first time. I started scratching at the correction fluid on the photo of the truck and suddenly the number-plate was legible. I looked at the photo of the three people watching me so intently and I wondered if one of them was the truck driver. Was he the one wearing King Gee khaki shorts and workboots? Was he waiting to see if I would live or die? Did he even get out of the truck? I knew from the police records that he hadn't stopped; that the motorcyclist had been the one to alert him to the carnage behind him. I had tried not to think about him over the years. Should I now? Was there anything to be gained? Do we have to confront those things before we move on, or is it just the past, to be left behind like I was that day, on the side of a road while the traffic moved quickly by?

Over the years, many people have asked me if I wish I hadn't been on the M4 that day. I can honestly say 'No'. If I could turn back the clock I would do it again. Not to the point of getting hit by the truck, no way. But I would live my life like I was living it then, like I'm living it now, in terms of being physically active and training. Accidents happen and that's part of life. I'm not caught up in that moment. I don't look back and say, 'Hey, I really wish I didn't ride my bike because my life would have been completely different.' Would it have been different if I hadn't been on this road that day? Absolutely. But let's go back to the cards I've been dealt. I'm just playing my hand the best that I can. Back then, I was living life to the full and absolutely loving it—and I'm doing the same thing now and have been ever since the accident. I'm not sure if I can add anything to that.

Cyclists ride their bikes on roads like the M4 every day. Some are riding to and from work; some are athletes training for triathlons or cycling events; some just want to keep fit and healthy. I've known people who've ridden their bikes along this same stretch of road and been hit by cars and killed. Just up there, on the exit ramp not far from where my accident occurred, a young cyclist called Matt Fisher, a lovely guy, married with two little girls, died. The point I am making is that things happen. I can't change what occurred twenty years ago, but I have tried not to let it change who I am or what I love to do—and that's sport. I'm not riding a bike competitively anymore—it's only going to be recreational—but I've been a professional athlete for a long time. Riding a bike or paddling or whatever—whatever—I've kept on going, essentially because the love I had for exercise pre-accident didn't change post-accident.

An interesting question was put to me recently that really did make me stop and think. Would I prevent my children from riding a bike on the M4? If I'm fortunate enough to have a child, or more than one, I would want to encourage them in whatever it was they had an interest in. If that happened to be exercise, I would encourage that, because that's part of a healthy lifestyle. If they wanted to pursue cycling as a form of recreation or as a competitive endeavour and they were at the age where they had the sense to ride a bike—which is well past the point of riding up and down the street with trainer wheels on—I would encourage them and be right there with them to support them. If that meant being on the freeway, I'd be more than happy to drive a car behind them to give them a bit more protection—you know, with the hazard lights on. If my son or daughter said, 'Hey Dad, you're being a bit silly, why don't you go and do something else, I've got this covered'—well, I guess I would have The Chat with them, but I still wouldn't want to wrap them in cotton wool.

If I have children, they will have to grow up with me in a wheelchair, knowing my story, seeing my challenges, but also my achievements.

CHAPTER TWO

ONE STEP AT A TIME

*'What John gives you is the way to deal with
those bad days better. That doesn't mean to say
bad days don't come'*
—Associate Professor John Yeo,
Royal North Shore Hospital

I spent the next three days in the ICU at Westmead basically
in a coma. I remember nothing of that time, even though my
medical records comment on my neurological state when I was
awake—whether I was orientated, confused or cooperative. I
was drifting in and out of semi-consciousness, heavily sedated
for the pain and shock. My condition had been stabilised, but
I was not out of the woods. I had been ventilated for most of
the time—a machine was helping me breathe and therefore
stay alive—and I had undergone numerous scans and tests
to ascertain the extent of the damage to my body, and the
operation on my broken right arm, in which pins and a plate
were inserted. All up I had seventeen broken bones.

My first memory after the accident is of the operating
theatre at Westmead. I remember looking up into the bright

lights. There was a nurse and I was trying to get her attention, wondering what had gone wrong. Then I lost consciousness again.

The doctors had warned my parents to prepare for the worst when I was admitted—I was not expected to live. The most positive comment on my records from Westmead appears on the discharge sheet prepared before I was airlifted to Royal North Shore, one of two Sydney hospitals with a spinal unit. In the top right-hand corner is the notation 'Discharged to survive'. I was off the critical list. I vaguely remember the helicopter journey and an odd feeling of excitement about my first chopper ride. Obviously the morphine had blocked out more than the excruciating pain.

I think we all have an invisible wall around us. We let in those people we love and care about (we speak of 'letting down our defences') and keep out those we don't. It's a protective barrier that guards us emotionally. Certainly mine was fully in place before the accident. But now my brick wall ... my invisible wall ... my confidence wall ... call it what you will ... had been shattered. I left the few remaining bricks at reception at RNS on the way in and picked them up again four months later on the way out. It would take years to rebuild my wall, and it would be a long and painful process.

The other thing I left at reception was my pride. If ever anything in your life teaches you humility, it is being in a spinal unit. Everything had changed. One minute I was invincible. I was a twenty-two-year-old thinking about football, running on the beach, having fun with girls, becoming a fireman. I was waiting for my application to sit the Metropolitan Fire Brigade test, keen to hear back about what the next step would be in this exciting career move, and wondering how I could successfully manage it and my football dream. I loved the notion of getting paid to keep fit and, you know, rescuing people—damsels in distress, cats up trees, all those sorts of romantic notions. The next minute, all of that was gone. My life had been turned on its head.

When I arrived at RNS, I was taken to Ward 6N ICU. I remember calling a nurse for the first time. My right arm was in a sling, but they'd left the buzzer by my left hand, which I could still use. The nurse who responded wrote on my chart that I was 'slightly confused but aware of what had happened'. She said I was 'anxious'. Absolutely. I was beyond anxious. When she came to my bed I said, 'I can't feel my legs.' I thought they'd been amputated and I was panicking. She reassured me my legs were still attached to my body by pulling away the sheet and showing me, and told me I had been in an accident. Then I passed out again.

I can't overstate the significance of this conversation, brief though it was. It was my first realisation that I had suffered more than a minor injury. I was holding on to life, but suddenly understanding that something major had happened to my legs, the limbs I treasured most. I will remember that moment, and the despair I felt, all my life.

I spent three days in ICU on level 6 before being moved to the spinal unit on level 7, where they have acute two-bed wards with specialist nurses and doctors. Effectively, it's an ICU for spinal patients. Members of my family and my girlfriend Michelle accompanied me the day I was moved, but I have no memory of their presence. Still, I'm grateful they were there. Spinal units are not the happiest of places, and if ever you need a supportive family or other people around you who care, that is the time.

From the time I entered Westmead, and all through my stay at RNS, Michelle was referred to as my fiancée. We weren't engaged, but she had to say we were to gain access to me. Hospitals are strict like that. Only the next of kin and close family members were allowed in the wards I suddenly found myself in. I loved Michelle. She was always the person I wanted to see the most and I never wanted her to go home. She visited me every day while I was in hospital, like clockwork, driving in from Tregear after work and driving back again after sitting with me for an hour or two. It took a huge physical and emotional toll on her and I will be eternally grateful for her devotion.

For the first few weeks at RNS I moved in and out of consciousness. I was in a drug-induced, very dopey state, and on oxygen the whole time. My family was very worried about me because when I was lucid I was emotional and kept telling them how much I loved them. 'We thought you were going to die,' my brother Marc told me later. I was also starting to realise the consequences of what had happened and where I was. Five days after arriving at RNS, I had a bad night. The nurse's entry at 6.30 pm on 4 July said: 'The patient was distressed and stated he found breathing difficult and thought he was going to die.' I was given 10 milligrams of Valium, an anti-anxiety drug and muscle relaxant, at 11 pm and again at 3.30 am, 'with good effect'. By the next evening my condition had improved. At 9 pm, I was 'being administered 60 per cent oxygen via a non-breathing mask'. I was stable.

Nights were always the worst times. I don't know whether it's the darkness, or the stillness, or the lack of distraction, or maybe your mind just thinks harder and deeper without the sun in the sky, but I always looked forward to the dawn.

I was scared in those early days. Really scared. I wasn't sure what was happening. I hadn't invited myself into this world, but suddenly I was part of the running of a spinal ward, meaning I was a patient and there was no conversation about whether I wanted to be there or not, or what my choice about anything might be, or what I wanted to happen. The job of the nurses was to get me out of there as efficiently and as professionally as possible. But I was twenty-two years old and I had just become independent. Suddenly that was cast aside. I had lost control over my life. Everything I had was gone. I was like a wild fox that had been roaming free and doing what it wanted to do and all of a sudden found itself trapped. I had a cage around me and I couldn't get away.

I understand why hospital staff monitor spinal patients closely. Some patients get depressed enough that they don't want to continue living. After I left hospital I met a guy who was in a wheelchair—the staff wanted me to come back to talk to him, to let him know that everything was going to be okay. He looked me in the eye and said, 'I am going to kill myself; it's just a matter of time. I'm going to do that.' And when he went home he did. He fixed a hose to the exhaust of his car, turned on the ignition and died. For him the pain of coping with such a dramatic change was so unbearable he chose not to live any longer. It was just too much. I have an appreciation of why some people call it a day. I also have an appreciation of why some others stay permanently medicated—they don't want to come back to reality because of how painful it is for them, both physically and psychologically. Dad said I was devastated by what had happened to me. 'I thought you wanted to end it if you could have found a way out,' he told me. But I didn't. Yes, I was devastated, but I had fought so hard to stay alive, I was so grateful to be alive, that I never contemplated taking my life.

That doesn't mean that I wasn't in a dark place during those early stages. I was. The doctors couldn't do anything for me, my parents couldn't do anything, Michelle couldn't do anything. No one could. Basically I was stuck in the spinal unit waiting for time to pass, 'to see how your recovery progresses, whether the nerves regenerate in your thoracic spine and what movement you get back'. I think waiting is the defining feature of a spinal ward. If you go into hospital with a broken arm, or see your doctor to get a prescription for the flu, you know you're going to be okay. The GP can give you medication or a specialist will set your broken arm. That's not the case in a spinal ward. They can give you drugs and all the rest of it to try to dull the pain, but in the end it's only time that reveals the ending to your story.

When I started to come to, it was a shock to realise what had actually happened. One of my earliest recollections is of saying to Dad, 'How's my bike?' So at first, obviously, I was thinking, 'This is a setback, everything is going to be okay, bones grow back together again, I know that, and I will get out of this place and play football again and everything will be fine.' But eventually I came to understand that things were not going to go back to how they were. I was in a spinal unit and there were wheelchairs moving up and down the corridor. *These people could not walk.* Battles raged within me about what life would be like in the future. It was a huge transition.

Every spinal patient is different—their injuries, their personalities and the way they look and interact with the world. I was what they call an incomplete paraplegic. My spinal cord was damaged at T12, around the same level as my belly button, but it was not severed. I was lucky, although my injuries held their own set of challenges. A guy in the other bed in my ward had broken his neck in a motorcycle accident and become a quadriplegic—he'd lost the use not only of his legs, but of his arms. Unlike me, he'd suffered no other injury, no broken bones or punctured lungs, just a slight laceration on his neck. I really felt for him—I heard his sadness, especially at night. And I heard his silences, too.

The pain I was suffering was of the highest level. Your spinal cord helps you to move and feel and, because mine was damaged rather than completely severed, I had hypersensitivity. I was in an immense amount of pain and thinking, like any person would, 'What can I do to get out of this?' I had never been burnt, but I had the sensation that a blowtorch was being run up and down my spine. Other parts of my body seemed to be screaming in unison with this dreadful sensation, and more than anything else I wanted to get out of the pain. It took a long time for that to go. The drugs helped. The good side is they block out the pain, but the downside is you are out of it. The medical staff try to get you off painkillers as quickly as possible, but I completely understand how people become addicted to medical drugs in that situation—anything to get away from that level of pain. If I had completely crushed or severed my spinal cord I would have had no movement or feeling beyond the point of injury, so I wouldn't have felt the pain I did—but I not only felt pain, I had hypersensitivity because there were still some connections.

I think the pain hitting me from all angles like that helped bring on a state of depression. All the negative emotions— anger, sadness and despair—came to the fore. As far as I am aware I was never given antidepressants. But it wasn't as if I could leave or go somewhere else either. I couldn't escape. So I learnt to retreat within myself. I became quiet and withdrawn and didn't want to communicate or engage with people or situations. I was as low as you could possibly go. Comments about depression start to appear in my records after about a month. It's clear I was being closely monitored, that staff were keeping a watch on my mental state and diligently passing on information from shift to shift.

They tried different types of beds to see whether one of them might alleviate the pain. (They didn't.) Orderlies had to come in and lift me—it took three of them—and turn me every couple of hours to prevent pressure sores from developing on my skin. This was most unpleasant, to put it mildly. At the time of the accident I sustained severe gravel rash over large parts of my face and body, not surprising given I was wearing only cycling pants, a cycling jersey, cycle shoes and a helmet called a skull cap, none of which afford much protection. Every time the orderlies lifted me, bits of my skin or the scabs would stick to the sheets.

The orderlies also put enemas up my bum. These were people I had never met before and they were doing *that* to me. They manually opened everyone's bowels in the morning, so you can imagine the stench. That was one of the main reasons I felt my pride had been left at reception. Other times the curtains around my bed opened and closed and a doctor would come in and introduce this person and that person, then they would talk *about* me in medical jargon that went completely over my head. I didn't know what they were saying. I felt like a book that was picked up and read whenever anyone chose to do so.

To add insult to injury they cut off my long hair, which had become matted and tangled. They said I had to have my hair cut, so I had my hair cut. There were lots of procedures I didn't like. I particularly hated the bird-bath. The nurse would bring a little bowl of warm water and a sponge. 'Mr Maclean, it's time for your bird-bath,' she'd say. I didn't like the nurse who did the bird-bath. I didn't want it but I had no choice. I was at the mercy of all these people—who all do an amazing job—but I didn't want to be in that situation.

One of the first conversations I recall is one with Marc, who was a trained nurse and probably understood more than anyone else in my family what I was going through—both physically and psychologically. 'It's a very serious accident,' he said. 'But I want you to look at this like it's a marathon. It's not a sprint. This is not going to be over and done with pretty quickly. It's going to take a while. So think about a marathon and keep on putting one foot in front of the other and you'll get to the finish line.' Marc had given me a sporting analogy which I could relate to. It was the best medicine anyone could have given me at the time and gave me a sense of hope which up until that moment I had not felt.

… keep on putting one foot in front of the other and you'll get to the finish line.

I can still remember every detail of the walls and curtains and cracks in the paintwork in my ward (which was right outside the nurses' station). That's the sort of thing that happens when you spend so long lying flat on your back. I could see North Sydney TAFE through the window, and I spent hours over the following weeks counting the number of bricks in the wall of the main building. I never did finish the count, but that didn't matter—it was a distraction, anything to keep from thinking about where I was and what I was feeling.

No one ever came in and said, 'You are a paraplegic and you are going to be in a wheelchair for the rest of your life.' That did not happen. But it did dawn on me that the things I loved to do most—walking along a beach, running in the bush, full-on football training—might be lost to me forever. I cried when I thought of this, but not often. The grieving I should have done then happened much later. I grew up in a family that didn't express much emotion. Dad would say, 'Boys don't cry. Be a brave little soldier.' I had taken those words to heart over the years, so I blocked out my feelings in RNS. I didn't process them or grieve like I should have, but I wasn't that sort of person then. I was a brave little soldier. When the sadness became more than I could bear I withdrew into myself.

As the cold, hard reality of my situation fully dawned on me, I confronted Michelle and offered her an exit from our relationship. Although we had been together for two years, and I looked forward to her daily visits more than anything else, what sort of life could I offer her? I first met Michelle in high school—we were in the same year. I noticed her because she was so good-looking, but she was more interested in the older guys then. Later, when I was playing for the Penrith Panthers, I saw her at the disco at the football club. She was with her boyfriend, but I asked her to dance anyway. Then some other guy started to make a move on her. 'Best you not do that, buddy,' I told him. A bit of pushing and shoving took place, and I was prepared to take it outside. No punches were thrown but I was ready to do whatever I needed to do. That's how I connected with her and she became my girlfriend.

How could I fight for her now? I was flat out fighting for myself. How could I stand up for her, on the dance floor or anywhere else? 'You should meet someone else,' I told her quite early on, when we were alone in the ward one day, or at least in my half of it. 'I can't hold your hand and walk with you along the beach. I want you to go and meet someone and do those things.' Her family told her the same thing. 'John is not going to be able to run again and do those types of things and maybe it's time for you to move on,' her dad said. They said it out of love for her and I respect them for that. But Michelle was tenacious and had strength of spirit and bravado and she stayed. I was her boyfriend and she was going to stand by me. 'Don't be silly, John, I want to stay with you,' she said, crying. 'None of this makes any difference. I want to be with you.'

I had lots of visitors in hospital, which I was sometimes up for and sometimes not. But I always appreciated it that people made the trip. My family—Dad, Mum, Marc and his wife Anne, and my sister Marion—all stood by me, showing their love and concern. I have never felt closer to them than during this time of my life. My mates came in too, trying to cheer me up with jokes and stories about what was happening in their world. I received lots of letters from the kids at Bennett Road, and from the teachers and parents.

And then there was Johnno, John Young. He came every Sunday, usually with his girlfriend Gail, who's now his wife and the mother of their two great kids, Chris and Rae. John was a front-rower in our football team, 190 centimetres tall and about 115 kilograms, so he was quite the unit. He is one of those rare characters who have an exuberance, an effervescent take on life. I had known him for about eighteen months. We weren't best friends at that time, but as the months went by and the visitor numbers dropped off, as they inevitably do, Johnno was one of the people who kept coming. He'd heard about the accident from our football coach at training the day after it happened. 'It was a big shock to everyone,' he told me. 'A lot of people were really upset about it.'

On reflection it must have been confronting for many of my visitors, including Johnno—a strapping guy who revelled in the physical challenges of his life, both in his work as a welder and in his sport—to come into a spinal unit and become aware of some of the more severe cases, like the quadriplegics who could only move their heads. The majority of patients in spinal units are men, which says something about our risk-taking behaviour, I guess. Johnno believed it was his job to be a supportive friend and do what he could to help. It was much easier for me to be positive when he was around. He was just that sort of person—he exuded the good things about life. He was always up, always happy, always setting the example that life was about living it, that we all should grab it by the throat and jump in feet first.

One person who never turned up was the truck driver who'd mowed me down. I really expected him to visit me. In fact, I was waiting for him. If I were in his position I would have had to, for the sake of my conscience. That's how I was raised. If the shoe had been on the other foot, I would have gone to the hospital, explained it was an accident and if the timing was right I would have said, 'I'm sorry. I didn't intentionally run into you.' I don't think I would have yelled or screamed or cried if he'd come in. I just wanted to hear those words and I would have said, 'Thanks for coming.' But he never came, and I put it to the back of my mind, along with many of the other emotions I was unconsciously storing away. I can't say I've thought about him often over the years—I don't think I allowed myself to or believed that it would have done any good—but there is something in that old saying, 'You don't want to die not knowing.' He was unfinished business.

I hit rock bottom in those first eight weeks. The good news was I had nowhere to go but up. They say that about spinal patients—that it's necessary we understand what we're facing. While it's true that some people do walk out of spinal units, many others don't. The best thing for me about hitting the bottom was that every little achievement became a milestone. I began to appreciate the small improvements, and that made a big difference later on. I was looking for things to hold onto. As time went by, what I wanted most was hope. Hope that I would feel better. Hope that my nerves would regenerate. Hope that I would one day walk again. One person who threw me a lifeline was our family doctor, Dr Atif Gabrael. I had been a patient of his since I was a child and he knew me well. 'Don't worry, John,' he said during a visit, in that low, authoritative tone that GPs spend years mastering. 'One day you'll be bigger, stronger and faster than ever before.' He didn't make false promises. He wasn't specific about his prognosis. He just made me feel I would move on, and I would get better. Those words were music to my ears.

Coming off the drugs was now something I wanted to do. One day a nurse came in and told me, 'We are gradually going to take you off the morphine.' I said, 'I've played football, I can take a hit, so let's go cold turkey.' So that's what happened—and I was introduced to another level of discomfort. The pain was heightened again. But the good thing about going cold turkey was I could get the tubes taken out of me and make some form of progress.

About seven weeks after the accident, on 18 August, life took a turn for the better. After a visit from my doctor, Professor Thomas Taylor, I was given the all-clear to shower on a trolley and to start to sit up, slowly, but sit up nonetheless. 'John is in very good spirits after this news' was the comment on my chart. Showering on a trolley meant no more bird-baths. It meant I was lifted from my bed onto a trolley with plastic straps and wheeled into the shower recess in the bathroom in my ward. I felt water spraying over my body for the first time in almost two months. It was a wonderful, exquisite experience. I absolutely loved it.

Sitting up was a different matter altogether. After eight weeks on my back my circulation wasn't as effective as it used to be. As they started gradually raising the head of the bed I began to feel really dizzy—but there was me being competitive, saying, 'Let's crank it up and get up there straightaway.' I paid for that.

After a few days they could get the bed-head right up without me feeling dizzy, and that meant my introduction to a wheelchair. Suddenly I was making progress. I was moved to a general ward and began to regain some sense of independence. But like life itself, it was not all smooth sailing. The gastric tube by which I'd been fed for so long was removed. The first few times I tried real food I threw up, but eventually my stomach got back to normal.

Now I was upright I could also go to the toilet by myself. I saw myself in the mirror for the first time—and my self-image was shattered in an instant. No longer was a cocky 22-year-old lad with long blond hair looking back at me; I didn't recognise the person I saw. I had lots of scarring on my face, my skin was sallow in places and grey in others, I was gaunt and hollow-cheeked. My hair was short. I had lost so much weight and muscle tone that bones were protruding everywhere. I stopped short and did a double take. I felt ill. I thought, 'I'm in a wheelchair, I've got scars on my face. Am I going to end up on my own?' This was absolutely the bottom of the hill. I had a lot of climbing to do before I could leave hospital and kick-start my new life.

I have always been a goal-oriented person. I believe it's important to set goals and to strive to achieve them. After the accident my first goal was to survive; my second was to get out of the pain I was in; my third was to get the tubes out of my body; my fourth goal was to get out of the bed. Each incremental achievement was a step towards making my own way again. I wanted to get outside, to smell the fresh air and to get out of the hospital environment. I wanted my freedom.

I vowed never to feel sorry for myself again—and I never have.

I mentioned earlier that no one had said what my future held. The medical staff had been careful to make no predictions. They can't. They say it takes about two years before you know exactly what movement you will get back after a spinal injury— and I was clinging to the hope that I would regain the use of my legs. I would run again. I would work harder than anyone else and I would make it happen.

Moving into a general ward was a life-changing experience, not only because it was the first time I saw the toll the accident had taken on my physical appearance but also because it gave me a sobering dose of reality about where I stood in the world of spinal patients. There were four beds in my new ward and the other three guys were much worse off than I was. They were all quadriplegics. I could still move my upper body and they couldn't. I felt sorry for those guys and I almost felt guilty, guilty because I was able to move my arms and I could dress myself, guilty because I was in a room with three people who could not, who required assistance for everything. So what did that give me? It gave me a sense of hope—that, you know, I'm very fortunate and I'm very lucky—and I guess from that point on there was a shift in the way I was thinking. How could I wallow in self-pity when I looked at these guys? I vowed never to feel sorry for myself again—and I never have.

I had turned an important corner. I wasn't in the home straight—in fact I was only at the starting blocks—but at least I was on the road to recovery and regaining my independence. I had started rebuilding myself. I was eating and drinking and putting on weight. And I was being taught to look after myself. Part of that meant self-catheterising. Previously, I'd had an indwelling catheter, which is a tube that goes inside the penis into the bladder. A fluid-holding balloon held it in place and the tube ran down the side of the bed and carried the urine into a bag. Because I couldn't void myself, I had to learn to self-catheterise four times a day or every six hours. I had to use Lubrifax—or something else water-soluble—to insert a syringe that contained xylocaine gel into the eye of my penis;

this numbed the area. I then gently fed the catheter in. Once it was in place the urine would run from the bladder into a dish. Another vital component of my health care regime was looking after my bowels. I had to go to the bathroom with a rubber glove and some Lubrifax, insert my finger in a circular motion and manually remove the faeces. I'm not explaining these procedures for any other reason than it's important to understand the full picture at this stage. I had been forced to accept changes to my body that I could never have imagined in my wildest nightmare.

Moving into the general ward was like getting a job and going to work. There was a routine. In the early stages, I concentrated on getting my right hand working again; the all-important radial nerve had been damaged when I broke my arm. The physiotherapists made up a special splint with fishing line so I could move my fingers. I had to wait for the nerve to regenerate, and thank goodness it did. Eventually I regained the full use of my hand. In the early stages, as part of my occupational therapy they used to give me things to do like taking a nut off a bolt and putting it back on again, working on getting dexterity back in my fingers.

I would also wheel down to the hospital's hydrotherapy pool. It took a while because the pool was over the other side of the hospital. I wheeled through an underground tunnel, then made my way into the changing room, where I would put on my swimmers and transfer into a PVC chair so I could go down the ramp and into the water. The physiotherapist put a flotation device on me made of the shiny bladders from wine casks; they were covered in a cheesecloth-type fabric so they didn't slip. I loved being in the water, the weightlessness and the sense of freedom it gave me. But I wasn't swimming laps straightaway. It took a long time to build myself up to that. Eventually I managed to swim 25 metres, which was as big an achievement then as swimming the English Channel ten years later.

The staff at RNS were amazing. I think the longer I was there the more I appreciated each and every one them. They were hard taskmasters but they were doing their best to assist everyone in the best way they could. I remember the physiotherapist called Debbie. I was on the gymnastic mats in my tracksuit pants and she told me to get on my knees and try to crawl. I had some movement in my left leg and foot, but she was still evaluating what muscles I had control over and what I didn't. She'd gently push me and I would fall over and get back on my knees again. I thought, 'Why is Debbie pushing me over?' But she was just seeing whether my balance was out and what she needed to work on with me. I thought, 'I used to play football, so how hard must it be for other patients who are not sports-minded?'

It was during a physiotherapy session that I wet myself. It was a highlight of my life; the implications were massive. Doing leg extensions with my left leg one day, my bladder just relaxed and let go. Without doubt it was one of my happiest experiences in hospital. I went back to the ward, had a quick shower, changed my clothes and wheeled down to the hospital chapel, which sits near the entrance to the main hospital building. 'Thanks very much,' I said, to anyone who might be listening. 'This is amazing. Thank you so much.' Some spinal patients never recover the use of the muscles that allow them to control their bladder and bowel. It was a sign of hope, hope that I was improving and that I would continue to do so. I am not a particularly religious person but I did turn to God in those early days. My brother Marc is devoted to his faith. He would sit by my bed and talk in tongues with his hands on my body. He believes in that sort of healing. I was ready to try anything, to believe anything that might help or aid my recovery. Although I didn't (and don't) altogether dismiss the power of religion or religious belief, at the time it was more that I could use all the help I could get.

Rehabilitation was like having been reborn. That's the best way I can find to describe it. I had to learn to crawl again. I had to learn to get in and out of bed and to use my right arm. I had to learn good hygiene techniques. I had to learn to dress myself and to use a wheelchair. I had to re-learn a lot of things I'd never imagined I'd ever have to think about again, and learn a whole lot of new things that I'd never imagined at all.

I felt fragile, too, which was another new experience. The hospital had become my nest, and even though I was keen to test my wings I needed to feel safe, too. My first outing was with Michelle, her girlfriend Jenny and Jenny's boyfriend John. They took me to Centennial Park for a picnic. I remember it so vividly, how beautiful it was seeing the trees and the grass, eating chicken and salad under the blue sky and smelling the fresh air. I have always loved being outside and I believe my time in hospital helped me to truly connect with nature. Nature has a calming influence on me and will for the rest of my life. On the way back they bought me a rum and raisin ice-cream, my favourite flavour—it was absolutely delicious. Back in my room again I went straight to bed and straight to sleep. Fatigue was a big factor in those early days, which I guess was understandable given what my body had been through.

Like a young bird I ventured a little further from the nest each time. My next outing was to Michelle's parents' place for lunch. Michelle picked me up and I can remember how long the process of getting into her car took. I used the sliding board to get from the wheelchair into the passenger seat, and I felt every bump in the road as she drove me to Tregear. I was still recovering from my injuries and I felt enormously apprehensive about those bumps. We had snapper for lunch, and by then I was exhausted. I slept on her parents' bed for an hour or two before Michelle took me back to the hospital.

A lot of things were going on for me at the time, not only medically speaking. There was also a fair bit happening in my head. My self-esteem had taken a battering and so had my confidence. I was asking myself, 'What's my life going to look like when I leave here?' I was in the process of rebuilding my wall. I was adapting to my physical challenges. I had to learn how to push a chair manually and do things like wheel-stands so I could get up and down gutters. I had to learn how to negotiate a bus with a bunch of other people in wheelchairs on an RNS social outing we went on one day. I had to learn about accessible bathrooms. It was like, 'How do I feel about that?' And I didn't like it. I mean, I liked the idea of getting out of the hospital, but I didn't like the idea of being seen in a wheelchair. It was about body image and the way that people looked at me. I didn't feel equal any more. It would take a while before I finally felt comfortable in my own skin again.

When the day came to leave RNS, I was determined to fulfil a promise I'd made to myself after I'd moved into the general ward and life had started looking more promising. I said, 'I will walk out of the spinal unit.' And I did, with the aid of Canadian crutches—the sort that have a clasp around the forearm and a hand-grip for more stability—and a steely resolve that helped me endure the slow trip along the length of the seventh floor to the elevator, through the automatic front entrance doors to the hospital, up the rise and past the chapel to where Dad had parked the car. It was a huge effort. Dad pushed a wheelchair beside me the whole way, just in case I needed it. It was certainly a case of slow and steady wins the race. I paused as I left that hospital, mentally picking up my pride and the few bricks left from my invisible wall that I'd left at reception four months earlier. I got into the car and didn't look back. I was utterly exhausted.

CHAPTER THREE

POSITIVE PEOPLE

'When we get together, it's all positive. Life is
good, it's too short to be negative'
—JOHN YOUNG, BEST MATE

September, 2008: So much has happened since I was discharged from RNS on 25 October 1988 that it would be easy to forget some of the details about the four months I spent there. That's why I've returned today. I've always found that being in a place helps jog my memory and unlock feelings long since buried. At the hospital's request I've been back twice during these past years to visit spinal injury patients, to speak to them about their fears and their hopes for the future and try as best I could to reassure them they could find their way again. But I've never sat in the ward or reminisced. I don't feel nervous or apprehensive about going inside, but I am glad I'm revisiting the experience, not reliving it.

Nothing much seems to have changed. The automatic glass doors at the front entrance glide open just as they did twenty years ago. The lifts are just as painfully slow as they inch their way from floor to floor. Even the public notices on the walls seem the same, although the dates have obviously changed. Time seems to have stood still at RNS—but maybe that's just what older hospitals are like.

I haven't made an appointment to see anyone today, but in spinal units you don't really need a calling card. A wheelchair is identification enough. I'm confident they will be pleased to see me because I have gone on to live my life. I'm not saying this makes me better than anyone else, it's just that I never gave up—and I think the people who work here like to see former patients who have gone on to achieve their dreams, whatever those dreams might have been.

The spinal unit is still on the seventh floor. As I wheel out of the lift and around the corner to begin my journey down the long, winding corridor to the wards at the other end, a wall of framed photographs greets me. Some are faded, others hanging a little crooked on their hooks, but it doesn't matter. They deliver an important message. They are pictures of former spinal patients doing things—sport mainly—basketball, wheelchair racing, tennis. People in spinal units need inspiration to get up and get going. They need hope that life will go on, that they will find a place for themselves in a world that will never be the same again. It helps them to know that others have travelled the same path and made a go of it.

Everyone needs a role model. One of mine is Associate Professor John Yeo. He ran the spinal unit at RNS for almost three decades before retiring recently, and the advice and friendship he gave me while I was a patient here was invaluable. I still see him and his lovely wife Joy regularly—usually over a home-cooked dinner at their house—and he is one of those rare men whose company inspires me to be a better person. John Yeo has snow-white hair and a quiet, considered tone that oozes wisdom and commands respect. When I was his patient he was conducting various research projects into spinal cord injury but he also had a deep insight into the mindset of the people he treated. 'Sometimes the miracle is not what you want,' he'd say, referring to the dream of all spinal patients that life will return to the way it was before their injury. 'It might be a different miracle.' He means the miracle of living; that you go on to meet your challenges and live with them as opposed to overcoming them. He believes that this is possible for every patient if they are prepared to share their journey with others—family or special friends. If you are on your own it is a harder road. I will always be grateful I crossed paths with him.

As I wheel down the corridor memories come flooding back. The scene is all too familiar—and so is that hospital smell, a combination of disinfectant and raw human emotion, a smell unlike any other. 'John Maclean, isn't it?' The person belonging to this voice is familiar to me too. His name is Speedy—at least that's what he's always been called—and when I was a patient he was a volunteer. Some time during the intervening years he has found his way onto the staff roster. We talk about sport and old acquaintances. I ask if it's okay to see the nursing unit manager and maybe have a look around. He takes me further down the corridor and into the nurses' station to meet Wendy Brown, who immediately extends her hand in welcome. She is wearing hospital-issue blue pants and a blue shirt and her hair is tied back off her face. She exudes a quiet confidence and a no-nonsense manner that I warm to straight away. A special breed of nurse works in a spinal unit. They say you need to be part larrikin, part sensitive soul. I thank my lucky stars for each and every one of them. They do an amazing job and I am testament to their dedication and unswerving commitment. I have not met Wendy before, but I feel I know her already.

I surround myself with positive people who enrich my life and who make me want to be a better person.

She takes me into the acute ward directly outside the nurses' station. It's like a flashback has occurred: 'I have a sense of being here before. This is the room. My bed was over there and look, there's North Sydney TAFE.' Those thought-deadening bricks are still embedded in the facing wall. There are thousands—no wonder I never finished the count. The floor is quiet at the moment. My old half of the room is empty, so we move closer to the window, where the view is exactly as I remember it. I ask Wendy about her work and her interaction with the patients. 'I don't know how it was for you, John, but I find that nights are tough for patients and we spend a lot of time talking.' I agree. Despair and darkness seem to go hand in hand. Still, what I remember most is the excruciating pain, that sensation of a blowtorch being run up and down my spine. It's now two decades since I experienced the full brunt of it, but I don't think the memory will ever dull. 'You would have been experiencing neuropathic pain,' Wendy nods. 'It's basically where messages are trying to get to your brain but the transmission is not quite happening. So you get altered hypersensitivity. It's not actual pain, but it's real.'

I've brought my medical records with me. Wendy is keen to go through them to see who was nursing me at the time.

Although staff turnover in any ward, in any hospital, is high, some members of staff stay for long periods or go off and come back again, especially in specialist areas like spinal units. It's possible, just possible, that some of the people who nursed me are still around. As she flicks through the pages I point out the references to depression that start appearing about a month into my stay. 'We worry more about the ones that aren't losing it a bit,' she explains. 'There is going to be a time when it hits and it hits some harder than others. It's an appropriate reaction. I think people need to see the negatives up front, because it *is* bad. It's important that someone in that situation knows that it's okay to grieve, it's okay to be angry, to think that their world is crashing down because every improvement they make after that is like, "Okay, I've got this far today, tomorrow I'm going to do this." It's a stepping-stone. You need the bad to create the good.'

Wendy scans my medical records the way I read sports results. There is always a story behind the statistics if you know the code that allows you to read between the lines. 'Sarah's still here,' she says, pointing to a particular page. 'That's her handwriting. You may have been one of the first guys she nursed. She's English. She's working today actually. You might recognise her.' At that moment, Sarah walks in. I do recognise her. She has a fair English complexion and blonde-tipped hair. 'I'm still here in the same uniform,' she laughs. 'I'd only just flown over from the UK when I started here.' I remember Sarah—she tried valiantly to make me more comfortable in bed, which wasn't an easy job given the pain ricocheting around my body like an echo in the Grand Canyon. She tried pillows and different beds, anything she could think of to ease the constant discomfort. 'Thanks for trying,' I say. 'I really appreciated it.'

The nurses were the people I spoke to most. There was also a social worker called Helen who came to see me from time to time. They call them psych liaisons now, but their role is still the same, watching out for the mental health of patients as they ride their emotional highs and lows. I'm sure the visits from Helen coincided with concerns expressed by the nurses. I didn't talk to her about my feelings much, though. We used to talk about ice-cream and gelato, everything else really. But I did talk to the nurses, especially at night. Wendy is right. That's when I was most honest. On 17 July 1988, less than three weeks after being admitted to RNS, I started contemplating the future. A notation in my medical records signals this shift in my mood: 'A restless night, wanting to talk about his present condition and future prognosis. Was reassured and explanations given, but very anxious.' Sitting here in the exact spot I had that conversation, I remember that feeling of panicked anxiety. I wanted answers which no one could give me. I wanted to hear that everything would be all right, that I would walk out of the hospital and pull on my rugby boots and run again. But no one could say that. I don't remember quizzing Sarah about it, but I could be wrong. At night I wasn't looking at a nurse's face. I was concentrating more on the pitch of her voice and the words she was saying and the words she wasn't saying, too. I never knew that unspoken words could be so important.

After my chat with Sarah, Wendy guides me down the corridor towards the general ward. Along the way we pass the visitors' lounge, where I can't help but notice a distraught-looking young woman who paces up and down the room before disappearing into an acute two-bed ward. An older woman— her mother or mother-in-law, I guess—sits there with tear-stained cheeks and swollen red eyes, and an older man, maybe her husband, stands bolt upright, stony-faced, with his hands jammed deep in his pockets. Was it like that for my family? Did they sit in those very chairs in the early days and cry too? Did they wonder how life would unfold for me and what the future could possibly hold? Did they pray they were asleep and would wake soon and realise it was all just a nightmare?

I never gave up.

I can't say exactly what it is that makes some spinal unit patients pick up the pieces of their lives and move on, or what it is that makes others want to give up. I do know that every brick of the wall I had built to protect myself came tumbling down when I entered this building and I had to start from scratch. Before the accident I was able to walk down the street and feel really comfortable in the skin I was in—but four months later I could only get about in a wheelchair. I felt different in every way. I struggled, I really did, in terms of self-confidence, self-worth and body image. I had to find myself again—and that took a long while. Coming back to RNS makes me realise just how far I have come.

I believe that adjusting my thinking helped. I know that as spinal unit patients go I am blessed. I can get around on crutches for a short distance, I can use my upper body, I am not brain damaged, I can go to the toilet and I can have an intimate relationship with a woman. In spinal units it's all relative. I have slept in the same ward for months with men who could only move their heads. I choose not to think about what I lost. I don't think I have that right. The way I live my life now is to be grateful for all the things that I have—and there are many.

I surround myself with positive people who enrich my life and who make me want to be a better person. My whole mindset has developed from that dark space I found myself falling into in hospital and all the dark times that followed. I do believe there was a purpose to it, and I have tried to understand it and apply it to my daily life. I refuse to feel sorry about any part of my life—and that attitude started here.

I regularly get requests from people to speak to family members who have suddenly found themselves in a wheelchair. I'm always happy to oblige, but I always ask first whether the person has requested it. If they haven't, if it's the idea of a well-meaning family, there's no point. I believe in the old saying that the master appears when the student is ready. I'm not saying that I'm a master of any sort, it's just that such conversations are pointless unless the person has reached a stage where *he or she wants* to talk to another person in a wheelchair. I know this from personal experience—timing is everything.

Today as I look at the family in the visitors' lounge, I know they are not ready to make a connection with me, not even eye contact. One day maybe, but not today, not yet. They are at the beginning of a very personal journey, and it will take time before they are ready to reach out. At this point it's a wait-and-see game, as it is for most in the early days. 'Even to this day no one will say what sensation a person will get back,' Wendy comments. 'Normally what you've got after two years is what you'll have to work with, but you can't be definite. We've sent people home who were incomplete paraplegics and they've come back in with the aid of a stick, even without one. Then there are others who have never walked or never got any more function back and that's because of their injury. Some know. If there is definitely no chance—the spinal cord is absolutely severed—we might say something. But normally, no, we don't make predictions.'

It is time to leave. The general ward is in the middle of a shift change and it's not a great time to be intruding on their routine. Nurses are experienced at goodbyes. They say them all the time. Down at reception I give Wendy a heartfelt hug. Then she turns on her heel and walks back down the corridor, into the lift to the seventh floor and those patients who are waiting for her, listening out for her footsteps up the corridor just as I would have been doing.

Wheeling out of RNS today is a whole lot easier than when I struggled out on those Canadian crutches so many years ago. It's a whole lot faster, too. I follow the same route as I did then, through the front entrance, up the concrete path, past the chapel and on to the parking area, and I cut the umbilical cord with the spinal unit that had been my home for four long months. I was so pleased to leave that day. While I'd felt safe and protected there, I was impatient to get on with my life.

Spinal unit patients usually go from RNS to the Moorong Spinal Unit in Ryde for further rehabilitation before they go home. It's a big step in the transition back to regular living. At Moorong patients learn to navigate the world with their wheelchairs. Wheelchair accessibility is such a vital issue that it helps to be properly prepared before tackling real-life situations. Catching public transport, using public toilets, accessing buildings and cafes are daily activities most adults don't think twice about. But like children learning to walk for the first time, people in wheelchairs must find out how to get around their homes, their communities and their cities.

When I left RNS, however, Moorong was fully booked, so I was sent to the Governor Phillip Special Hospital in Penrith instead. This hospital began operation in 1865 as the Nepean Cottage Hospital; in 1962 it became the Governor Phillip Special Hospital to provide special care to the chronically ill and aged, and in 1974 an 80-bed nursing home to provide care to the aged and the physically challenged. I can't remember how long I was scheduled to stay, but I was in for a big shock when I got there.

Today, as I pull up at the front entrance, I notice the signboard outside which says 'disturbed and confused older persons', with an arrow showing visitors where to go. I hadn't noticed this sign back then, but it doesn't really surprise me. The clean white façade and the manicured gardens still present a calmer, more serene image than what I experienced inside.

Back in 1988 the average patient was at least seventy-five years old. I was just twenty-two, uneasy at leaving the safety of RNS, where everything was accessible and safe, entering a geriatric hospital where everyone else was frail or had dementia, where people passed on. Leaving RNS meant, I thought, that I would regain some control over my life. But I soon realised that was not to be, at least not immediately. Dad helped settle me in and asked, 'What would you like for dinner?' I love charcoal chicken, potatoes and pumpkin, and I told him that's what I'd really like. But the matron had different ideas. 'No, you'll be eating with everyone else,' she said. And I thought, 'Okay, I'll have to toe the line'; it was almost like being back in primary school. We had powdered scrambled egg. To go from charcoal chicken to powdered scrambled egg didn't exactly bring a smile to my face. But worse was to come.

There were four beds in the ward I was in, but only two other patients, both dementia cases, I believe. As the night wore on, one of them was wandering around the room with his appendage hanging out of his pyjamas and the other was screaming incoherently. I got the sense that when people get older they revert back to their childhoods, and it really scared me. It gave me an insight into what life could look like, and why it is so important to enjoy the moments along the way. I began to think, 'You know what, don't have any regrets, John, because life is too short for that.'

I love movies. One of my all-time favourites is *Dead Poets Society*, in which Robin Williams plays English professor John Keating. When his students find his photo in an old yearbook, Keating uses the opportunity to deliver a very important message. 'They're not that different from you, are they?' he says, referring to the young men featured in the yearbook. 'Same haircuts. Full of hormones, just like you. Invincible, just like you feel. The world is their oyster. They believe they're destined for great things, just like many of you; their eyes are full of hope, just like you. Did they wait until it was too late to make their lives even one iota of what they were capable? Because, you see, gentlemen, these boys are now fertilising daffodils. But if you listen real close, you can hear them whisper their legacy to you. Go on, lean in. Listen, you hear it? *Carpe*, hear it? *Carpe, carpe diem*, seize the day, boys, make your lives extraordinary.'

I had not seen that movie before I was admitted to Governor Phillip Special Hospital. But when I did watch it a few years later it resonated strongly. *Dead Poets Society*, which was directed by the Australian Peter Weir, and my experience that night became inextricably linked. Today, I can't think of one without the other. Governor Phillip Special Hospital made me realise that I didn't want to grow old with regret about what I had achieved in my life—or what I had not—and the contribution I had made. *Carpe diem*. I wanted to seize the day.

I also thought during that disturbed night about my own mortality. How did I want to die? Certainly not on the side of the M4 after being hit by a truck, or in an ambulance speeding to hospital. Definitely not in a geriatric hospital, alone and confused in the middle of the night. Hopefully my deathbed will be very different. I'd like to be surrounded by my family and friends, people who love and care about me, who would hold my hand and I theirs. I'd like it to be a good death, where I leave this world at peace with what I have achieved and the relationships I have nurtured.

I slept badly when I slept at all that night. In the morning I pleaded with Dad, 'You've got to get me out of here. This is not right at all.' And to his everlasting credit Dad talked with hospital management and got me out that very afternoon. I was on my way back to the family home in Tregear.

CHAPTER FOUR

GIVING IT 100 PER CENT

'For me his mental resolve far exceeds his physical achievements. When he puts his mind to something he just locks it in'
—TRENT TAYLOR,
JOHN MACLEAN FOUNDATION

My childhood might be described by some as tragic—but I don't see it that way. I loved life during my childhood and have nothing to complain about. Over the years, however, I have come to explore the age-old question of nature versus nurture. Just how much did I learn from my parents and the environment I grew up in, and how formative were those factors in moulding the person I became? Were my personality and behaviour predetermined by the genes I inherited? Was I born this way? Certainly it was genes that were responsible for my blue eyes and my turn of speed. But I cannot discount the sum of the personal experiences that prompted me to confront my life and ultimately my fears.

I was born in the early hours of the morning on 27 May 1966 at Caringbah Hospital, near Cronulla, in Sydney's Sutherland

Shire, the youngest of three children. My dad, Alex Maclean, and my birth mother, Avril Maclean, were Scottish immigrants who'd come to Australia in July 1965, less than twelve months before I arrived on the scene. Unlike my brother Marc, three years older than me, and my sister Marion, two years older, I was conceived in Australia. My dad had been a policeman in Rutherglen, a small town outside Glasgow, by day and an entertainer by night. He was a singer when variety was entertainment's headline act; he also had a show on television for a while that made him something of a local celebrity. He had previously been married to Margaret, and they'd had three children, Don, Morag and Kenny. The marriage became troubled and finally broke down completely. Then Dad married 22-year-old Avril, and they decided to start over with a clean slate in Australia. Whether this was a good decision or a bad one is not for me to judge. But they were moving to the other side of the world, where they knew no one and had no family support to help raise their small children.

In other circumstances Avril may have found the strength and resilience to make a go of life in this new country. But the odds were stacked against her. According to her medical records Avril described her own childhood as 'unhappy', although it is noted that this view could be attributed to the depression which developed in her teens. By all accounts, she had a close relationship with her parents, my Grandma Elspeth and Grandpa Jack, on whom she greatly depended. She had only one sibling, her sister Meryl, who was a few years younger. Grandma Elspeth said Avril was overactive and vivacious but found it very hard to make friends. She was an average student but good at sport, an aptitude she passed on to her children. On leaving school she worked for three years as a tracer but left her job after being wrongly accused of theft.

It seems that at eighteen Avril's life began a downward spiral—she suffered a nervous breakdown and was admitted to Robroyston Psychiatric Centre in Glasgow, where she underwent electroconvulsive therapy (ECT), more commonly known as shock therapy. She was discharged a short while later, but at the age of nineteen was admitted to the Department of Psychological Medicine in Glasgow. A letter from a consultant psychiatrist at that time details her concern about putting on weight, and her apparent reliance on the amphetamine Dexedrine, a highly addictive stimulant. She'd started taking it after having her tonsils out some time earlier, and by now, whenever she stopped taking it she felt listless and depressed. The day before she was admitted she'd gone to Dunoon, a popular coastal resort, with the intention of killing herself. As far as I am aware, that was her first thought of self-harm. Nine months later she was diagnosed as 'suffering from a severe character disorder of a psychopathic nature'.

Dad wasn't aware of Avril's chequered medical history before they married, and it wasn't until they arrived in Australia that he began to realise the extent of her illness. Why he hadn't noticed anything wrong before that I don't know. Why her parents hadn't said anything to him I don't know either. That Dad had taken their sick daughter so far away was a source of conflict with his in-laws for years. In those early days he was working three jobs to pay the bills, including the rent on a house at Loftus, in Sydney's southern suburbs. Money was tight and they had not been in the country long enough to have established a social network or good relationships with neighbours. I cannot imagine a more difficult scenario for either of them. Then I was born. Adding a baby to an already stressful situation must have been like adding fuel to a fire.

For a time we moved to Medlow Bath, between Katoomba and Blackheath in the Blue Mountains, while Dad tried to obtain public housing. He had thought that living in a nice quiet area might do Avril good, but on 18 March 1967, when I was less than ten months old, she was admitted to Parramatta Psychiatric Centre and diagnosed with a serious illness called 'schizophrenic reaction'. There she underwent a course of fourteen ECT treatments and was prescribed other medication before being discharged into Dad's care three months later.

What happens to very young children when they are separated both physically and emotionally from their mother? If you asked my brother and sister, they would have different versions of the experience and the impact it had on them. I guess it depends a lot on how old you are and what memories you have stored up.

I don't recall ever feeling connected to my mother in any way. I can't remember her face, her smile, her smell, her cuddles or her voice, telling me in a hushed, gentle tone that she loved me. There's nothing at all. And that has been a big void in my life. What did it mean for me? I grew up looking for attention and affection and love in other ways. I thought, 'If I can excel at something I might be praised or recognised.' I tried to jump higher and run faster than anyone else so that someone might think, 'Johnnie's done good.' I love my father and I know he did his best bringing up three kids in difficult circumstances. He loved us, but it was a different love to a mother's love. It was more disciplined, more stiff upper lip and do the right thing, don't cry, don't swear, don't be disrespectful, try hard at school. We got belted, sure. Everyone did in those days. But I thank him for instilling the importance of respect.

Avril was in and out of psychiatric institutions for more than three years after that first admission to Parramatta. No sooner would she show signs of improvement than she'd hit the skids again. I don't think she ever kicked her reliance on Dexedrine, which she turned to regularly to make her feel better and to battle the depression that was never far from engulfing her. Ultimately it did her no good. It only contributed to her mood swings and fits of depression and aggression, her downward spiral of despair.

In August 1967 she was reported wandering around The Gap at Watson's Bay, a popular suicide spot in Sydney's eastern suburbs. She later told her medical officer she wished she'd jumped, as she 'was no good to her husband and children'. It wasn't the only time she found her way there. Three months later police took her back to Parramatta after she was found at The Gap again. She told the police she was confused and had undergone ECT recently but couldn't remember where.

In a desperate attempt to stabilise her health, Avril returned to Scotland to visit her family in 1968. Dad offered to take us all back permanently but he needed help with the fares. Avril's parents' response was that there wasn't much work in Glasgow so perhaps it was best she came alone. She returned to Sydney the following year, but any improvement to her mental state seems to have evaporated by the time her ship docked at Circular Quay. It was now 1969 and the marriage was under a great deal of strain. Dad was managing as best he could but he couldn't raise three young children and work at the same time.

In March 1967, shortly after Avril's first admission to Parramatta, Marc, Marion and I had been separately placed in the Dalmar Children's Homes. I was only a baby, not yet walking or talking. We were admitted and discharged six times over the next four years. I have no memory of being at Dalmar, but their records indicate they knew me well. 'John continues to be a loveable child, although mischievous,' they noted in February 1969. I think I was lucky to be so young. Not only do I not have any memories of that time, but younger children had greater supervision by adults and I suspect a greater chance of feeling loved. Marc, on the other hand, had largely to make his own way with children his own age, including the odd bully. We weren't together, so there wasn't even sibling solidarity to fall back on.

By late 1969 Avril's condition had worsened further. We had moved into a Housing Commission home at 9 Penguin Place, Tregear, and Marc, Marion and I had been discharged from Dalmar. But on 12 December, Dad called the police after Avril said she was going to give us tablets so we could 'go to God'. She was taken back to hospital, where a medical officer described her as 'aggressive, paranoid and thought disordered', displaying 'uncontrolled schizophrenic behaviour'.

I could go on—the medical records are nothing if not detailed. Suffice it to say things didn't improve. Ten months later, at 12.30 pm on 2 October 1970, Avril's body was found at the foot of the cliffs at The Gap. She had taken her own life some time late that morning. She was only twenty-nine.

A coroner's inquest was held later that year. A medical superintendent from Parramatta told the coroner Avril's 'illness was characterised by self-deprecating ideas and hallucinations. I gather that she quite frequently spoke of herself as being an unworthy person and at times said that "the voices" told her she should kill herself'. No one saw her jump but the coroner said the possibility of her falling accidentally was so remote it could be discounted; additionally, the severe fracturing of both ankles indicated she had landed feet first.

I call her Avril and not Mum because I never knew her. It would be thirty years before I properly mourned her loss. The most difficult page for me to read in her medical records was the one that included these words from a social worker in 1967: 'Mrs Maclean told sister she didn't mind the other children, but can't bear the baby, aged fourteen months.' That was me. I know she was sick. I also know she cared—and that is what is worth holding onto. There are entries in the records— notations made during her more lucid moments—chronicling her concern at how long we were spending in Dalmar. I have since been to her grave and been struck by how young she was, how briefly she lived and how much she missed out on.

Avril died because she didn't want to be a burden any longer and she didn't want to hurt us. I think she felt she had no other way out. Once I was clear about that I felt calmer—I had made peace with my mother. Forgiveness is powerful. Every person wants to love and be loved. I am no different. I can admit, though, that it took years before I could let a woman into my heart. First, I needed to feel comfortable in my own skin and figure out what it was about my life that wasn't working. But all that comes a little later in this story.

I didn't go to Avril's funeral—I was probably considered too young. I don't remember Dad explaining how she died. I think Marc told me many years later. He'd found out from our neighbour, who happened to be the person who retrieved her body from the rocks. What are the odds on that? He had been living next door to us for years.

Dad met Anne, whom I have always called Mum, in December 1970, at a New Year's Eve function at the Western Suburbs

Soccer Club in Five Dock. On their second date they collected us from Dalmar and took us on an outing to the zoo, so he was pretty upfront with her from the start about his family situation. I admire my dad for not giving us up for adoption. I think the Dalmar social worker asked the question of him at least once and he replied, 'That's not going to happen, these are my kids.' Anne had lived in foster homes herself and gone to boarding school, even though her mother was alive. She and Grandma Penny—that's what we called her mother—had a life-long complicated relationship.

Anne was 27 and Dad 43 when they married. They had lived together for three months before they tied the knot on 27 November 1971 at a little church in Rooty Hill. We children all went to the wedding. I was dressed in exactly the same shirt and tie as Marc and can be seen beaming from the wedding photographs. Three and a half weeks later, on 20 December 1971, just in time for Christmas, we were discharged from Dalmar for the last time.

I was rapt at being part of a proper family. I was old enough now to want to be just like any other kid. Now we had a mother, and that was pretty special, right? We were normal now. We had Christmas and we went on holidays and we used to go to the drive-in. We'd get in Dad's big Pontiac and drive to Penrith, where we'd line up in the parking lot with everyone else. I'd watch the movie until I fell asleep on the pillows on the back seat. Dad and Anne were working and we were a family.

That fibro-cement house in Tregear is the only family home I have known. It sits on a slight rise at the end of a cul-de-sac, but that is the only feature that distinguishes it from the other houses in the street. There are no brick houses here because this is not an area that can afford anything grander. Tregear is a small blue-collar suburb, 46 kilometres west of Sydney's central business district. It has two sets of traffic lights, a primary school, a preschool and a small shopping centre. It is part of the City of Blacktown, but is probably more often thought of as part of Mt Druitt.

Penguin Place was filled with children. The families who lived there had all moved in at the same time and we grew up together. When there was a game of cricket on, all the kids came out to play. We'd go down to the smash repair shop and get some ball-bearings and build billycarts. Sometimes, at night, we'd douse the wheels in petrol and light them up as we raced down the street. We were nicknamed 'the gutter rats', and we'd stay outside playing until it was dark. On Australia Day Mr Brown from number 6 would block off the street with witch's hats and we'd drag out our barbecues and have a big cook-up. Was it tough growing up here? No, this was the best street in the world.

I was fortunate enough to go to South Africa recently; while I was there I went to the township of Soweto. Large parts of Soweto have no running water, no toilets. Families struggle to put food on the table, if they even have a table. In comparison, our family was rich. We never wanted for clothes or a roof over our head. Dad had his regular job and Anne worked part-time as a sales assistant at a department store. We were able to put an extension on the house; we had a nice car and were heavily involved in the community. Looking back, I can't say we did it tough because we didn't.

I went to Tregear Primary School, like all the kids in the street. The older ones would take charge of the younger ones as we walked there with our schoolbags slung over our shoulders. Academia was not my strength—it wasn't something that came easily. Dad would often talk to me about the importance of knowing my times tables. When he came home from work he would get me doing them, and if I couldn't do them correctly, he would not be happy. Many years later I was talking to him at a Christmas function and said, 'Dad, why was it so important to you that I did my times tables?' He said, 'Son, because I wasn't any good at them and I wanted you to be.' 'Guess what, Dad?' I replied. 'I'm no good at them either!'

At school I didn't daydream about being a nuclear physicist, I'd be looking out the classroom window dreaming about sport, because that's what I was good at. I used to run around the perimeter of the grounds during lunch break, and sometimes I'd run home and raid the ceramic 50-cent coin-jar that sat on the dresser in Dad and Mum's bedroom. The round trip was about 5 kilometres, but I could get back before the bell went with enough time to spare to go to the shop near the school and buy lollies to share with my friends. Some people might say I had ants in my pants, but I just liked to move. My life was fluid. If I had been born in water, it wouldn't have been in a pond. It would have been in a river, where there was a strong, flowing current.

I got caught nicking those 50-cent pieces. Dad was head cleaner at Penrith Police Station at the time, and teed it up for me to get a bit of a lesson from the boys in blue at Mt Druitt. Here I was aged twelve, and Dad was putting me in the car and taking me to a police station! The sergeant who took me around the place said, 'If you do stuff that's wrong, here is what happens to you. You get fingerprinted, you will have a police record and you will go into a cell like this.' I was packing it! Dad said to me on the way home, 'If you continue to steal this is the life that you will live.'

I think I was basically a good kid. I wasn't shoplifting from supermarkets or milk bars. I wasn't out late at night and drinking alcohol and stealing cars and taking drugs. I wasn't interested in things like that. I was keeping fit and enjoying my life with a cool group of friends. But I am still glad that Dad took me to the police station and imparted that lesson via the sergeant. I was taught from an early age what was right and wrong. To this day, I respect my elders and I don't swear—and that comes from Dad.

Sport was what we did as a family. We were all involved. Dad always said it was a good way of meeting people and making friends. In winter I'd play rugby league and in summer I'd do Little Athletics. My Saturday mornings started with waking early. I'd watch cartoons—which I absolutely loved—and then go out and do whatever was scheduled for that day. I remember how it rained one weekend when I was seven and I couldn't play rugby league. I was devastated. It was the end of the world. 'What do you mean I can't put my boots on and play football?' I cried. That year my grandparents in Glasgow sent me a book for my birthday present—I was so disappointed it wasn't a football.

I don't care if you come last in every race as long as you give 100 per cent.

I was good at sport—and successful too. When I was in Year 6, I won the under-12 national championship in race-walking. The principal called me up in front of the whole school at assembly. He said: 'John was the best in New South Wales and then he won the national championship and now he is the best in the whole country.' I wanted to be the best that I could be and I was comfortable with that, but at the same time I felt very uncomfortable about being paraded in front of the whole school, being so publicly acknowledged.

I didn't think I was better than anyone else because of my win, but of course some kids thought I did. I found myself at the receiving end of comments like: 'He thinks he's better because he's the best in the country.' You know what kids are like—the 'cut down the tall poppy' syndrome. What I learnt from that experience was that it's better to fly under the radar. At sixteen I was named junior athlete of the year at Dunheved High School and I vividly remember refusing to be exposed to the whole school. I remained standing in line and I just wouldn't go up to receive my award.

There wasn't any expectation at home that I be the best. I wasn't expected to win. Dad would buy me a good pair of running shoes or whatever I needed and all he asked was that I give it 100 per cent. He was very clear about that. There was one occasion at Little Athletics, when I was twelve or thirteen, when Dad saw me in a race where I didn't give my all. He wasn't impressed. He gave me a couple of kicks up the bum, told me to pick up my gear—blocks, bag and shoes—and had a few words to me on the way home. 'I don't care if you come last in every race as long as you give 100 per cent,' Dad said. What he meant was that he went to work and didn't earn a lot of money but what he did have he spent on me, my brother and sister. He wanted us to appreciate that—and that meant us 'giving it our best'.

I took that lesson to heart. Whatever I do in sport or business—coaching and mentoring managers—or in other aspects of my life, I give it everything I have. I've been asked to sign a few things over the years—books, posters, T-shirts—and I always sign 'John Maclean 100%'. That goes way back to when I was that little kid who got his bum kicked at Little Athletics. Dad's philosophy was impregnated into my mind then and nothing has changed.

Marion was also talented at sports—she was terrific at softball and touch football—but it was Marc who was the star of the family. Academically he was smart, and he was good at rugby league football too. He was my hero.

Marc was seventeen when he did his HSC in 1980. His rigorous workload included physics and chemistry, which he found particularly difficult and stressful, on top of the HSC being stressful in itself. At the same time family tensions were building as he started forging his own identity and asserting his independence. Eventually things became so fraught that Marc left home. He failed the HSC, but in time he went on to study and became a nurse. In 1985 he married Anne and they moved to New Zealand in December 2001. They've got two children, Marcus and Jasmine. We keep in close touch, but I miss him.

When Marc left home Marion and I grew closer. I hadn't paid much attention to my sister up until then—we'd pretty much grown up not talking to each other—but Marc's absence threw us together. Even now we ring each other all the time, if only to say 'hello'. Not a week goes by that we don't speak.

Marion trained as an aerobics instructor (she later became a weight loss life coach), and in 1980 she met a lovely guy called Tony. They married and moved to the back of Tony's parents' place in Lethbridge Park, not far from Tregear. Tony is Italian and one of sixteen children, and Marion immersed herself in the whole Italian culture. She and Tony never had children. They separated after seven years of marriage and in 1999 she met Kerry. They married in 2001 and have one daughter, Alana, who was named after Dad (the 'Al' part is short for Alex), so I have three nephews and nieces now, who are just as important to me as my brother and sister.

CHAPTER FIVE

BEING MYSELF

'People love John, even when he was a young kid, because he's funny and he took life as he found it. He was always like that. What you see now is no different to how he was before the accident'

—MARC MACLEAN, BROTHER

I was sixteen when I left school after doing my school certificate in Year 10, the end of an unspectacular academic career. I wasn't sad about leaving, or concerned about what might lie ahead for me in the tight labour market of the day. My interests lay elsewhere—I was keen to chase my dream of being a professional rugby league player. Sport was my passion, and I had always believed it was my future.

In the meantime I found a job working for a Safeway supermarket, collecting empty shopping trolleys from the car park. I had to wear dark pants, a white shirt and red tie, and a red apron. I didn't know how to tie a tie at that stage (I'd never had to wear one, even in school) so I bought the kind with elastic attached that allowed me to just pull it over my head. A voice would boom out over the loudspeaker system, 'Service 40 to front end', which was code for 'John, get some more trolleys'. My record was fifty in one long, snaking line. If anyone needed evidence of my competitive nature or goal-setting tendencies they only needed to see the pride I took in beating each personal best and then setting a new trolley target.

Looking back, I suppose it was quite humbling. My friends' parents shopped there, and other people I knew, and there I was scrambling around the car park collecting trolleys. It wasn't what most young blokes aspired to when they left school, but at the same time it involved physical activity—running back and forth, pushing the combined weight of numerous trolleys— which has been a constant theme in my life. It was also doing an honest day's work for an honest day's pay, and that was not to be sneezed at either.

The Safeway job lasted about a year, then I joined a labour-hire agency that provided workers for builders and bricklayers. I'd ring up on a Monday morning and ask, 'What am I doing this week?' and then head off to wherever the job was, in any one of several different suburbs but never too far away. I was living at home and had bought my first car, a Holden Torana, which I was paying off. Some of my friends had moved out of home by then but it wasn't an option I gave much thought to, probably because I was on such a good wicket. My meals were cooked and my washing done for me, an ideal set-up for a young guy starting out in the world. I was keeping fit and loving my life—and that included always having a girl on the scene. I did casual work for the agency for a couple of years until I started playing for Penrith Panthers Rugby League Football Club, when they helped set me up with a job as a general assistant at York Primary School in Penrith, where my salary was about $15 000 a year. I wasn't going to get rich from it, but working school hours meant I was always available for training. From there I moved to a similar job at Bennett Road Primary School in St Clair, where I was working when I had the accident.

My career ambition was to become a fireman and play professional rugby league at the same time. The two, at least in my mind, fitted together perfectly. Firemen worked shifts, which would leave large parts of the day available for training. I was sure I could combine the two and juggle the hours. I had it all mapped out. I had been graded at Penrith, playing in the Under-23s team, or third grade. I had played about six games for the reserves in second grade and was gunning for a shot at the big time—the first grade team. Rugby league is a game of skill and brute strength, but it is also a game of chance. I was a winger. My greatest asset was my speed and where possible I used it.

> I've stuck true to who I am my whole life.

In 1986, Graham Murray, who went on to have a distinguished coaching career and retired only recently, took over as coach of my third grade team. I was nineteen at the time and pretty cocky. I'd had a great season, found I was faster than the guys playing first grade, and was looking to step up. Unfortunately Graham Murray and I didn't seem to click. I should also mention that David Bolton, a first grade assistant coach, had pulled me aside one day and put ideas in my head. He'd said, 'You have a lot of speed and the objective of this game is to put the ball over the try line, not to run it up and knock yourself out. So, when you see the opportunity, run around a few players and get yourself into space and accelerate and put the ball over the line.'

I took this advice, which proved my undoing, at least as far as my future at Penrith Panthers was concerned. But it also said something about my character and approach to life that I will never apologise for. My fall-out with Graham Murray happened on a game day. His instruction, to the best of my recollection, was to settle the play, which meant taking the ball into the forwards, where I would be tackled but the team would hold possession and set a play for the next attack. But I saw an opportunity and I went for it. I ran down the side of the field and almost scored a try, being caught just before the try line. Murray was very upset—he pulled me off the paddock and sat me on the bench: 'You listen to what *I* tell you!' I didn't get too many opportunities after that. Before the end of the season I was told my services were no longer required.

There are two sides to every story. Graham Murray was the coach and it was his game plan and I should have stuck to it. If I had, possibly I would have gone on to play rugby league football at the highest level. Who knows? But that's not the essence of who I am. It wasn't me. I backed myself and I don't have any regrets about it. I've stuck true to who I am my whole life. Later on, after the accident, when I felt the whole world was closing in on me, that inner drive to excel and achieve, to go after what I wanted, was what helped me survive and move forward. It became my most valuable personal asset and that's why I don't look back now and think about what might have been.

... eighty per cent of success is rocking up. I know that to be true. You just need to have the courage to get into the game.

Many people have been successful because they stuck with what they knew and believed in—and not only in sporting circles. Transport magnate Lindsay Fox, for example, didn't do well at school, but he bought one truck, then another and another, until he had built up the largest trucking business in the country. I think it's important to say to people, 'Be yourself, don't try to be somebody else.' The other thing I've learned along the way is that you are not going to get on with everybody. Some people are always going to rub each other the wrong way, and that's okay. Lots of other footballers had a good relationship with Graham Murray and went on to successful careers. I just wasn't one of them. But I wasn't going to throw a wobbly and sit at home and hate the world. I kept on going. It reminds me of the Rolling Stones song, 'You Can't Always Get What You Want'. Those lyrics still ring true.

It broke my dad's heart, though, and he held on to that moment in time. 'You had the opportunity to play first grade football if you'd just listened to Graham Murray,' he used to say. He wanted me to toe the line. But I wasn't like that. We had a next-door neighbour—his name was Bert—who I used to visit in hospital when he was dying. 'Time waits for no man, John,' he said. He was right. Life moves forward. And unless you want to be left behind you should move with it.

I'm not saying to anyone, especially children, 'Don't listen to the coach.' If it were my son or daughter involved in a team sport, I'd tell them, 'The coach is there to coach, so listen.' When there is a falling-out it is the coach who stays and the player who leaves. But there are always other teams to play for, other goals to chase. If my son or daughter wanted to continue playing in a team despite some conflict, I'd probably say, 'Well, hey, maybe you need to toe the line because Dad didn't. If you listen to the coach you might get a chance of playing more often.' But I would also encourage that child to 'back yourself, and believe in yourself'. I guess it's a case of finding the right balance. I love that old saying, that eighty per cent of success is rocking up. I know that to be true. You just need to have the courage to get into the game.

CHAPTER SIX

SETTING GOALS

*'In my view there are three types of people:
those who make things happen, those who
let things happen, and those who say, "What
happened", and John is one of those people who
makes things happen'*
—Ross Cochrane, CEO Express Data

No one ever said, 'John, you will never walk again.' For a long while I believed I would. I truly thought it was only a matter of time before the effort I had invested into rebuilding my broken body would pay dividends and somehow, miraculously, I would resuscitate my legs and go on to live the life I had dreamed of as a child. It was not to be. But the next few years were not spent in vain.

I went on to learn the lessons of a lifetime. I discovered the true nature of friendship with my mate John Young, who I now call my brother; I married Michelle, the beautiful woman who stood by me in hospital, and then lost her because our timing was not quite right, or the lack of chemistry between us that I thought would change never did; I reconnected with my family, especially Dad, who went from being a parent finally free of his responsibilities to a father caring for a dependent son again; and I started getting fit and healthy—lifting weights, swimming, paddling—I loved doing this and it helped me rediscover my sense of self.

This was not the miracle I'd prayed for in hospital, but it was a miracle nonetheless. Associate Professor John Yeo was right. I was sharing the journey and accepting that I needed help, and life was definitely, absolutely, worth living.

I had plenty of incentives to get myself walking again. I didn't want to be in a wheelchair. I didn't like being in a wheelchair. And if the truth be known, my self-confidence had taken more of a hit than I let on to anyone, even myself, particularly when I saw my reflection in the mirror that first time. We all have a perception of ourselves—the way we look, the way we move, the way we interact with the world around us—and for that to be so dramatically altered in such a short time was a really confronting experience. Walking again, or at least trying to, gave me hope and purpose.

I hated the way people looked at me in a wheelchair. I felt I could hear their minds ticking over and that inevitable, unspoken question on the tips of their tongues: 'I wonder what happened to you?' People do it without thinking. It's a reflex reaction. A young, otherwise healthy young man in a wheelchair equals a tragic accident. I didn't know what was worse, the quizzical, double-take stare or the sad face brimming with sympathy and concern. Four months earlier I had been able to walk down the street feeling really comfortable in my skin. Now I was wheeling. I felt different within myself and I struggled with that for a long time.

I had taken so many things for granted and one of them, which really surprised me, was being tall. In a wheelchair I was suddenly shorter than everyone else. It may seem a minor point, but I know now why they say short men develop inferiority complexes and short women feel compelled to wear skyscraper heels. I know why kids want to grow taller—they want to be able to see over the counter! Having everyone look down at me all the time generated a very negative image—more so in my mind than in anyone else's—and to this day I don't like being in crowds or around a lot of people. I think that's because I don't like having to look up all the time.

But the central issue for me post-accident was not being seen as equal. For a long time I felt that way. Some people might say it was my issue, the personal challenge of facing up to what had happened and to the fact that I would probably be in a wheelchair for the rest of my life. There's some merit to that point of view, but I don't think it was the only factor.

The looks I'd get from people and the fact that I was sitting down low in a wheelchair were bad enough. But the way society labels physically challenged people didn't help either. Suddenly I was called 'disabled'—and I don't feel comfortable with that word. Disabled means non-functioning, and I function very ably. I dissociated myself from that word a long time ago and am confident enough now to stand up against its use. It makes me cringe. It says, quite clearly, 'You are less than others, move aside.' Well, do you know what? I am absolutely equal. I am not going to the side. I am going forward.

I take a stand on this wherever I can, most recently in 2008 when I declined a $2000 scholarship for Athletes with a

Disability from the NSW Institute of Sport designed to offset the training costs of preparing for the Beijing Paralympic Games because it carried the word 'disabled' in its title. I was granted a different scholarship worth $500, but I believe the $1500 loss of income was a small price to pay for a principle I feel so strongly about. I intend being a lifelong advocate for dissociating the word from humanity. I don't want people in wheelchairs seeing themselves as being less than other people and, most of all, I don't want children growing up believing it either, whether they are physically challenged or not.

So what would I prefer to be called instead? 'Physically challenged' or 'people with a level of need'—I'm comfortable with those terms.

From small things big things grow, both good and bad. I am personally acquainted with the issues for people with special needs, and I believe it's important to give back to your community where you can, to use your experience and knowledge to help others who are travelling after you. There is nothing better than working with young kids in wheelchairs and seeing the hope in their faces when you talk about what they can do in their lives, as opposed to what they can't.

To overcome the gnawing feeling of inequality that stayed with me for so long I needed to set some goals and achieve something extraordinary. But the first thing I needed was to get back to Tregear. I would be lying if I said I had a triumphant homecoming. The disastrous night at Governor Phillip Special Hospital had done little to lift my spirits or instil much confidence in what lay ahead. But I was glad to be home. The sense of freedom and normality it gave me was a much-needed tonic, and there was something very comforting about being back in the same bedroom, in the same house, in the same street, with familiar neighbours who had known me most of my life. I felt safe—and that was important, because I also felt very vulnerable.

I have often thought we treat our older generations badly and underestimate the richness they can bring to our lives if we just open the door to them. I was lucky, because there were a number of older people in the street and in those early days after my return home they were always around during the day, when Dad, Mum, Michelle and my friends were at work. Mr Baker was our next-door neighbour and not very well at the time. He would sit on his porch and watch me battle up and down the cul-de-sac on my crutches. I'd set little goals, striving to reach a certain pole one day and another, a little further on, the next. It wasn't easy. My biggest issue was the burning sensation in my right foot and trying to drag my legs through after I'd inched the crutches forward. My left leg was stronger than my right, so I placed my weight on it, but I still had to pull my whole body through for the next tentative step. Another neighbour, Mr Brown, would come with me sometimes, and I'd struggle from his house to the bottom of the street and back. Eventually I got down to one crutch and two laps of the street. To this day I don't know which of us it punished more.

My relationship with my family changed, too. I believed my dad softened a lot after my accident. He looked after me all over again, just like a new parent nurturing and caring for a newborn. Not only was he running me around all over the place before I could get a driver's licence again, but he cooked for me and made sure I had a glass of stout every night before I went to bed, the stout which every Scotsman believes is the elixir of the gods and the cure to all aches and ailments. He gave me as much love as he could. I think my suffering touched him in a way that nothing else had. He would massage my feet and legs and offer words of encouragement and when I was down, really down, he would sit on the side of my bed and try not to cry with me, although sometimes we shed a few tears together. My dad had led an interesting life. His passion was singing, and although he once sold out the Sydney Opera House with his show 'Scotch On The Rocks', his musical career didn't take off in the way he hoped it would. Dad was a stoic person and I think I learned a lot from him about never giving up on life. Of all his children I think I enjoyed the best he had to offer as a parent. The accident was the main reason for that. He had no expectations of me after I was hit by the truck, so the sporting success I enjoyed later on was an exciting turn of fate. It gave him some proud moments he had never expected.

I was sharing the journey and accepting that I needed help, and life was definitely, absolutely, worth living.

As the youngest child I think Mum always felt a greater connection to me, perhaps because I had no memory of our life before she became part of our family. Anne was good to me and she loved and cared for me throughout my childhood, so my achievements post-accident were important to her. Marc had moved away a long while before the accident, but he was also supportive when I returned home. So was Marion. I spent a lot of time with Marion over the next few years and grew to rely on her.

What must a parent think when their child has a catastrophic accident that leaves them in a wheelchair? Did Dad and Mum wonder if I would recover enough to be independent again? And what of my state of mind? I am often asked about that: 'Just what is it that got you through? Why were you able to pick up the pieces of your life and move forward and others can't?' I believe the answer lies in who I am, who I always was. It's a combination of my drive to achieve and my upbringing. It goes back to little Johnnie wanting to jump higher and run faster than anyone else to be noticed and loved for doing that. I was also fortunate with my injuries. Because I am an incomplete paraplegic, I can stand for short periods of time, I have some feeling in my legs, I can manage my bodily functions. That's a lot to be grateful for and I remind myself of that every single day.

I didn't use the wheelchair much in the beginning. I thought I could exercise and train my legs to do without it, that if I succumbed to using it I would lose the impetus to get rid of it. I am single-minded and focused when I set my mind to something, and rebuilding the strength in my wasted body was paramount. I was on a mission. Not only did I use the street as a training ground, but I devised a strict rehabilitation program that I was convinced would get me back on my feet. Dad started work early in the morning at Penrith Police Station; he'd come home to drive me to the hydrotherapy pool attached to Governor Phillip Special Hospital, then on to Ron Oxley's gym in Penrith, where I worked out for a couple of hours. Then he'd bring me home for lunch and an afternoon nap. I was sleeping a lot in those early days, at least twelve hours a night and another three to four hours during the day. It was like that for the first three years. It's not that unusual in cases like mine, because I was still recovering from what I had gone through, but the sheer exertion of doing without the wheelchair was responsible for a large part of my fatigue. It was a battle between mind and body, and I think both paid a price in those early days.

I also started training in the garage in the backyard, which we had turned into a makeshift gym. I had no shortage of training partners but John Young was the one who stuck. Other friends would burn out after a while but Johnno never threw in the towel. In the beginning I thought he would go the way of the others and told him so. 'Thanks, it's great to have someone to train with but you'll burn out and I'll see you later,' I warned him. 'I'll burn out, will I?' he replied. 'We'll see about that.' His shift finished at 3 pm so he had time to train after work. We made benches and adapted equipment because money was tight, and it developed into a full-on, out-of-control competition. Whatever we did—weight lifting, bench presses, chin-ups, sit-ups—we egged each other on.

Johnno's way of connecting and communicating with me when I left hospital was, 'Let's go. We're going to take this on and we're going to get the best that we can get for you.' He knew I believed I would walk again and he wanted to help me make that dream come true. We thought if we stayed healthy and positive we could do it together. That's the love of a friend for another friend. He took me on like you take on a demanding job and I am so lucky to have him in my life. If you asked him today when it was he realised I wouldn't walk again he'd say, 'I still hope John will walk again one day. With science something will be developed and he'll walk back into that hospital.'

One day Johnno went to pick up some fibreglass resin for work and spotted a two-man touring kayak, or TK2. This looked like something he and I could do together, he thought, so he suggested it that very afternoon. Within a fortnight we'd gone halves in a kayak and were trying it out in the hydrotherapy pool at Governor Phillip Special Hospital. By then I had developed a friendship with a guy called Ched Towns, who worked at the pool as an assistant to the physiotherapist.

Ched was married with two beautiful kids and was training for the 1998 Seoul Paralympics—he'd been selected to compete in javelin. He was visually impaired, which seemed an odd pairing of sport and athlete. Ched became a great friend and helped me a lot in those early days. It was Ched who allowed us to use the warm pool when Johnno and I first started trying to balance ourselves in the kayak, which must have scared the pants off the 80-year-olds who were doing their aquarobic classes at the same time. I'm sure they ended up laughing just as much as we did, for we really struggled to find our balance and spent most of the time tipping into the water as opposed to staying upright in the boat. My right foot spasmed frequently and shook a lot, but eventually we found our equilibrium. The kayak was important because it gradually moved my indoor exercise regime—pool and backyard gym—outside and into nature, more specifically the majestic Nepean River.

Ched and I started training together too, first at the local swimming pool doing laps, but when that became hazardous because people often jumped into our lanes we relocated to the Penrith Lakes. By now I had a driver's licence again, so I'd pick Ched up after work and we'd drive down together. Then he'd carry me into the water. We'd tie ourselves together with a Velcro leg rope and head off. Swimming in the lakes gave me a whole new appreciation of the water, especially for the weightlessness I felt and the sense of connection to nature. There was also the satisfaction of realising that two people with different levels of need—a para and a blinky—could complement each other so well.

Around the same time Johnno and I tackled the Nepean River with our new kayak. The first time we went for a really long paddle, only a few weeks after we'd bought the boat, we headed off up the Nepean River towards Warragamba after Johnno finished work, intending to head back once we reached a certain point. We'd left too late in the day, however. Almost as soon as we turned around it was pitch black. After a brisk stint of paddling in the dark, my backside and legs began to hurt badly, so we stopped and sat on a rock on the bank for a while, thinking, 'This is more comfortable than that stinking boat.'

Then we headed off again. It was only about 16 kilometres back but somehow it felt as if we weren't getting anywhere. Johnno started singing a line from this old fishing song he'd learnt as a kid, 'What I want is a proper cup of coffee made in a proper coffee pot', over and over. He was driving me nuts, and probably himself as well, but he kept on singing because he knew we needed a distraction, even an irritating one, to take our minds off the situation. It was freezing, and so dark we could barely see our paddles. I was a little bit scared. So was Johnno, I think, although neither of us would admit it. It's not the sort of thing blokes own up to. I cursed our foolishness and hoped nothing went wrong because we were in such an inaccessible area, at least by road.

As we rounded the next bend we were relieved to see the light on in the captain's cabin of the paddlewheeler *Nepean Belle*, the floating restaurant. We started paddling as hard as

.we could in its direction. We were like a couple of exhausted horses that had been out all day but could still muster the energy to gallop the last kilometre when they saw the home yard. Unfortunately we hit a submerged log and capsized. Then the *Nepean Belle*'s lights were turned out and once again we were in total darkness.

I swam ashore and Johnno dragged the kayak towards me until he could stand and turn it upside down to tip the water out. It was hard to find somewhere with a secure-enough foothold to get back in the boat, and he was hoping he wouldn't tread on a bit of old bone or a piece of broken glass. I hated being thrust back into the darkness, but we made it back to our starting point not long after that. I was never so glad to see the freeway bridge over the river or to get out of a boat in my life.

I didn't know it at the time, but each experience on the water with Johnno, however challenging, was invaluable in building up my confidence. Bit by bit I was rebuilding my invisible wall and regaining my I-can-do-anything attitude. I wasn't there yet, but slowly, slowly, it was coming back.

Buoyed by the successful outcome of our adventure up the Nepean, we decided to enter the Hawkesbury Canoe Classic, a 111-kilometre kayak race on the Hawkesbury River, colloquially known as Madness by Moonlight because you set off at dusk and paddle all night. The race starts in Windsor and finishes in Brooklyn and is Australia's second-longest canoe event after the 404-kilometre Red Cross Murray Marathon. With Michelle and Gail as our support crew we started the race a little wobbly, hoping we wouldn't embarrass ourselves by falling into the water within sight of the start line, but soon found our rhythm and out of a field of about 100 we finished twelfth. I was ecstatic—we'd been competing against able-bodied people. I was involved again in competitive sport and felt more energised than I had in ages.

Johnno and I competed in the Hawkesbury Canoe Classic a number of times. Our best result was second in our category, and we would have won if we'd made better strategic decisions. More significantly, though, one year we didn't finish. Our boat sank and we had three letters recorded against our names in the record books—DNF, standing for 'did not finish'. Sometimes a person's failures are just as influential as their successes and Johnno and I both hated that our names appeared alongside those letters. Years later, when I wanted to call it a day during a particularly gruelling event, I remembered how bad I felt after that kayak race with Johnno. The letters DNF spurred me on.

I felt safe with Johnno. Sure, he helped me rebuild my physical stature and upper-body strength, but it was more than that. Tregear is a pretty hard, blue-collar area and when we went to the local club in our late teens it was not uncommon for a fight to break out. That doesn't mean I was in the middle of it, but I was always confident I could look after myself. That changed after the accident, I felt vulnerable. When I was with Johnno, however, I always felt secure. We'd often joke that if a fight broke out I would jump on Johnno's back and get a higher leverage point to throw a few punches.

It was a different scenario entirely with Michelle. When we first hooked up at the disco in Penrith and a guy put the moves on her, I had been willing and able to take the confrontation outside. I was prepared to fight for her, defend her. Now I was in a wheelchair I didn't feel that was possible. If anyone said something offensive there was nothing I could do. That's really why I didn't want to go out and socialise—I felt inadequate.

Michelle thought I'd changed in those first twelve months. I was less confident.

My first Christmas after the accident was a very dark time. We were at Marion and her husband Tony's place in Penrith. Perhaps it was the contrast with the jollity of the season, but whatever it was, the reality of my situation suddenly weighed heavily on my shoulders. I never got angry or violent or swore at anyone in a visible show of emotion; I carried my anger and grief neatly tucked away inside. I became withdrawn and quiet, and for those who knew me it was a sure sign that not all was well with my world. I'm still like that today, although not much bothers me anymore. I think once you have hit rock bottom you appreciate the small things in life. That was a positive outcome from those dark days; they gave me a relative sense of good fortune.

Michelle and I became engaged in March 1989, three months after that Christmas. There wasn't a bended-knee proposal on my part, it just sort of happened during the course of a conversation. Michelle said, 'We've been going out for a while now and it would be nice to get engaged.' I agreed. I loved Michelle; she was a beautiful person. It made sense, even though in hindsight it was far too early a stage of my recovery to commit myself to anyone. How could I? I was training most of the day, didn't have a job to support her or any children we might have, and I wasn't comfortable enough to go out with her at night in public.

It didn't occur to me that Michelle and I were on very different journeys. She loved me and wanted the whole package: a husband, a house and a family. She wanted to live in her local community, near her mum and dad, and raise some children. I loved her too, but more than anything I wanted to prove myself. I wanted to walk again, and I thought I could make that happen through hard work. Even when I accepted the inevitable, that I would be in a wheelchair for the rest of my life, my drive to excel was no less diminished. There was a fire in my belly propelling me to go out and achieve something in my life. I didn't know exactly what that entailed or where it would take me, but I wasn't ready to settle down in Tregear, or anywhere else for that matter—at least not just yet—and that altered the chemistry between us.

It took about two years, but I finally accepted that I wouldn't walk again. It was before Michelle and I got married and I was still living at home with Mum and Dad. I had given it 100 per cent. I had pushed myself beyond all reasonable limits and refused to use the wheelchair, but in the end I came to the conclusion I was only harming myself, knocking myself out when the energy I was expending could best be directed elsewhere.

I had discovered that paraplegia is not something you beat. I don't want to discourage other spinal cord patients who are waiting and hoping that the nerves in their bodies will regenerate, for, as I've said before, each case is different and it depends on your injuries. For me, though, it was time to face the cold, hard truth. I was in my bedroom with Dad when I first said it out loud: 'I'm trying as hard as I can but nothing is happening.' Dad looked at me as only a parent can, and I got the sense he knew that I was not going to get any better. It was a cathartic moment. He looked at me and I cried: big, heartfelt tears. Dad was misty-eyed too, although he held it together.

I gave him a hug and then he said, 'But look how far you've come. Now, how far can you go?'

Accepting the wheelchair was a tough reality check—but it certainly made life easier. Suddenly I could get around without superhuman effort, and the fatigue that had dogged me like a black cloud since the accident seemed to lift. I still liked a kip during the day but I wasn't completely blown away—not like when I was struggling with the crutches and using up all my energy just moving my body.

It was an important psychological step as well. Letting go of one dream allowed me to start thinking about another. I won't say it was easy, because it wasn't. I'd never pictured myself being in a wheelchair for the rest of my life and it was an image that would take some getting used to. But when I let go of the false hope of walking again, I turned a corner, I moved forward. That was a valuable lesson. Sometimes life is what it is and no amount of striving will change things. People who understand that don't get stuck in the moment. That day in my bedroom with my father by my side and an uncertain future staring me in the face, I learnt that I cannot control everything in life, and I shouldn't try.

Our wedding took place on 9 September 1990. Michelle and I were both twenty-four. An old friend from childhood, Colin Thomas, who is still a good mate today, was best man and Johnno and Ched were groomsmen. Michelle wore a beautiful white dress that made her look like an angel, and I donned a tuxedo for the first time in my life. I was excited about getting married and looked forward to being with her. The fabric that held us together didn't start unravelling until a year or so later, but at that moment I very much wanted to commit myself to her and our future together.

Communication in a relationship or at work or in any aspect of life that involves people is absolutely critical.

We moved into my parents' place afterwards. We hadn't lived together beforehand, but not many people did at the time. Dad and Mum retired to the South Coast and sold the house to me. It was a generous act pending settlement of the court case over my accident.

I received a sum of money from the court case that helped me make a fresh start. Michelle and I sold the house in Tregear and paid my parents back the money I owed them and bought another place in Penrith. It was a step up for us. Ched and his wife Judy had introduced us to the street and they lived not far away. I loved the area and the house was a stone's throw from the Nepean River, which became an important landscape for me as I continued training with Johnno. I'm not sure about Michelle though. In some ways I think she was happier in Tregear, but maybe that's because our relationship seemed on more solid ground there than it did in Penrith.

During the court case I reconnected with Professor John Yeo. I went to see him at his rooms at RNS a short time afterwards to talk about employment opportunities. 'I would like to help kids in wheelchairs. Is there any job that you could recommend or suggest where I could be involved at that level?' I asked. John Yeo had started a program with Errol Hyde, a great guy who was also a paraplegic, following a motorcycle accident. The program was called the Awareness and Prevention Program—later renamed Spinesafe. At the time there were about three hundred spinal cord injuries in Australia each year and the theory was to send us out into schools to educate kids about the fragility of the spinal cord and provide awareness of how to protect it, with the view of reducing the number of accidents. I was offered a job with the program not long after that.

As part of my training I went out with some of the other lecturers and watched how they did their talks. I was given a few props, like a model of the spine, and helmets and splints that quadriplegics use, but at the end of the day I needed my wits more than anything else. I was really nervous at the beginning, fronting up to a whole lot of kids I didn't know, trying to keep some semblance of order while teaching them a few things about anatomy at the same time. But I grew to enjoy it. I liked the little kids most because they had no inhibitions. 'How do you go to the toilet?' was one of their favourite questions. 'How do you drive a car?' They really zoomed in on the basics as they tried to process how a person in a wheelchair navigates ordinary, everyday tasks. The older girls in high school were a different species altogether. I was reasonably confident, but still sometimes taken aback by their very personal line of questioning. 'Can you have sex?' they'd say, straight up. I was being hit on by a bunch of eighteen-year-old girls! (I have to admit it did wonders for my ego, though.)

Gradually I developed my own style of presentation. I enjoyed visiting the primary schools most, I think because it allowed me to be a kid again myself. It was really hard initially because if I didn't tune into those kids quickly they would eat me alive. Literally, they would just tune out—and once they were gone, so was I. Every lecturer had their trump card and mine was that I could always pick out the boy who was the class clown and destined to cause me the most grief, probably because I identified with him so strongly. I'd bring him up to the front of the stage and include him in the presentation. I'd say, 'You're such a good kid I want you to sit right here next to me. I want you to sit up nice and straight because you're my number one man.' The other kids loved it because he'd be the kid who was normally stuck in the corner.

I learnt how to communicate with those kids and how to engage them, which was really effective in terms of their learning. I had it down pat. I would introduce a conversation but would leave out parts of the sentence, which they loved to finish. 'Hi, my name's John and I've broken my ...' and I would stick my hand around my back and they'd all yell out 'Back!' 'That's right. What's in the middle of the back? It starts with an S.' They'd yell out 'Spine!' 'Okay, what's in the middle of the spine? It's called a spinal something, can someone help me out?' And they'd scream out 'Spinal cord!' I made them part of the presentation so when they left I knew they understood everything because I had embedded it into their little minds. After a few months I was presenting to a whole school on my own, which the teachers loved.

We also gave presentations to traffic offender programs. These usually comprised people who had registered high-range DUI (driving under the influence) readings and gone in front of a judge who'd said, 'You have the choice of attending this program and having your sentence reduced, or taking the maximum penalty.' Obviously people would go and do these courses, but the majority of them didn't want to be there. We'd give them a harsher type of talk, the nuts and bolts of what takes place after a serious accident. It was more personal than the stuff you'd share with kids and I found it more confronting, but after a while I started to relax and just be me and it fell into place.

A car came with the job and I started travelling all around New South Wales, meeting and talking with people from different walks of life. I loved it. I was being paid to learn to communicate and although I didn't know it at the time I was serving an apprenticeship. Today as I make my living talking to business managers and mentoring executives around the world I often reflect on the time I spent in those classrooms. It's about making a connection with people. You just need to know your audience.

> ## Some goals you achieve, others you don't. In the end, it doesn't matter. The key is to keep on setting them.

I worked with Spinesafe for about six years before finally calling it quits. It shifted the course of my life and I will always be grateful for that opportunity.

Life at home, however, was not so great. The more I reconnected with the world the more Michelle and I seemed to drift apart. I was working during the day, then training into the evening with my mates in the gym out the back. Before that I used to at least cook dinner at night, but now Michelle did everything. She worked, shopped, cleaned the house and cooked all the meals. There were times when she'd say 'Dinner's ready' and I'd tell her, 'I haven't finished my training yet, I'll be in after that.' I admit I was too focused on myself and my dreams to recognise it.

Towards the end of 1994, three and a half years after we were married, Michelle said to me, 'I want a change for a while.' It was all very amicable. Marion and Tony came to help her move her things. Her brother came over too, and her mum and dad. We never had a real fight about separating or a direct conversation about why it was happening. Years later Michelle told me: 'I didn't want to go, I just wanted you to appreciate what I did for you.' She was waiting and hoping that I would pick up the phone and say, 'Hey, Michelle, I love you and I realise all the stuff that you do and I want you to come back.' I didn't know she wanted me to do that. And that's one of the lessons that I learnt from that experience. Communication in a relationship or at work or in any aspect of life that involves people is absolutely critical. Because she didn't say it, I thought, 'Well, okay, she wants to have a bit of a break and move on. What I need to do is organise things and keep going.'

By that stage I'd had some profound experiences—good and bad—that had given me a different take on life. The night at Governor Phillip Special Hospital had scared the pants off me. I had a glimpse into what it's like for lots of people who have dementia and who are elderly and going through the whole palliative care process. I looked at myself after that and thought, 'I don't want to spend another day, let alone thirty years, with someone who is going to look back on that time and say they wished they weren't there.' So when Michelle said she wanted a break I thought, 'If you're not happy, I'd much prefer for you to go and be happy somewhere else rather than have you stay here and say to me you've been unhappy for a day, let alone years. I'd prefer for you to go on and meet someone who was perfect for you and have a great life.'

In fairness, I didn't have the maturity to articulate what I was thinking even to myself, let alone to Michelle. So nothing was ever said. She assumed the phone would ring, but I never made the call. Instead, I spoke to Home Care, who sent someone over to mow the lawns and do the washing and cleaning while I kept on going to work and busting myself in the gym.

The fact is I did appreciate Michelle and everything she did for me, but our marriage had been built on an unstable foundation. We have spoken about it since and she agrees with me. We wanted different things. I had this fire in my belly telling me I had to do something with my life, and I wasn't going to be content until I found out what it was I was chasing. I felt restless and driven, just as I did looking out the classroom window as a kid.

My favourite athlete is Muhammad Ali, the greatest boxer the world has ever known and, I believe, the greatest athlete of all time. 'What keeps me going is goals,' he once said. I know exactly what he meant. Goals have defined my life. My first goal after the accident was to survive, the next to walk again and feel equal and comfortable in my own skin. Some goals you achieve, others you don't. In the end, it doesn't matter. The key is to keep on setting them. Ali also said, 'It's a lack of faith that makes people afraid of meeting challenges, and I believed in myself.' It's like we were reading from the same script. Despite everything that had happened in my life I never lost my belief in myself. It wavered after the accident and for a while later on, but it never died. It is perhaps the greatest gift I was given and one I urge people to try to find within themselves. If you can't believe in yourself, who will believe in you?

At the time of my accident I was cross-training for the Nepean Triathlon, one of the biggest events of its kind in the country, attracting about a thousand competitors. I had competed in both 1986 and 1987 and enjoyed the physical challenge it presented, although I wasn't a star contender, mostly because of my poor performance in the swimming leg. The first year I competed I did breaststroke, not freestyle. Penrith has a large, committed triathlon community, somewhat like a sporting family. The city nestles at the foot of the Blue Mountains and its wide, open spaces gives those interested in the sport plenty of opportunity to train. The event comprises a 1-kilometre swim, 40-kilometre bike ride and 12-kilometre run. It is quite challenging because the course includes some very steep hills as it winds its way up from the Nepean River.

I never lost my belief in myself. It is perhaps the greatest gift I was given and one I urge people to try to find within themselves. If you can't believe in yourself, who will believe in you?

In 1994—six years after being hit by the truck—I decided I should finish what I'd set out to do before the accident and compete in that triathlon again. Early in the year I had seen a hand-cycle, which is a three-wheel bicycle hand-operated by pedals set at chest height. The seat sits much lower, slung between the two back wheels, than it does on a traditional racing bike; the single wheel is at the front. A heavy piece of equipment weighing about 25 kilograms, it was a revelation to me. Now I could start competing in triathlons, or at least try to. I mentioned the idea to Johnno, who gave a nod of satisfied approval, and I bought one soon after. I started training in earnest and loved it from the outset. My training partners rode their bikes while I hand-cycled.

As the day of the triathlon drew near, I suffered a crisis of confidence. At that time no other wheelchair athlete in Australia had competed in this event, or any other triathlon for that matter. I said to Johnno, 'I'll do it, but I'll do it the day before anyone else.' I thought that might take the pressure off. While I was fitter and more comfortable in my skin than I had been straight after the accident, I still cringed at the looks I attracted in the street, and certainly at the looks I imagined I would get competing with more than a thousand able-bodied athletes. 'What are you talking about?' Johnno said, with the look I knew not to argue with. 'You're going to do the race with me and everyone else on the day. And that's all there is to it.' There was no further discussion. I entered the race.

There is a song called 'Two Little Boys', written by Edward Madden but recorded by Australian singer Rolf Harris, which typifies the relationship between Johnno and me. We often joke about it privately. It's about two little boys called Joe and Jack who are best friends growing up, helping each other through their scrapes and mishaps. When they are old enough they go off to war, where Joe is wounded on the battlefield and lies dying. But Jack does not forget his friend:

Did you think I would leave you dying
When there's room on my horse for two?
Climb up here, Joe, we'll soon be flying

Back to the ranks so blue.
Do you know, Joe, I'm all a-tremble.
Perhaps it's the battle's noise;
But I think it's that I remember
When we were two little boys.

Race day came around and I was nervous. Johnno piggybacked me into the water for the start of the swimming leg. Johnno was a faster swimmer than me at the time and he had to wait for me for something like four minutes after he finished. When he saw me approaching the finishing line he ducked down in the water and I swam right onto his shoulders and wrapped my arms around his neck; he lifted me out of the water and carried me up the hill to where my hand-cycle was waiting.

The sight of us created some attention and someone on the microphone said, 'Ladies and gentlemen, we have a guy in a wheelchair competing today', and people were clapping. I thought, 'Oh, okay.' But I still didn't feel very comfortable. Johnno helped me onto the hand-cycle for the bike leg. 'You're okay?' he asked. 'Yep,' I said. 'All right, I'll see you at the finish line.' Other competitors were going by very quickly. The hand-cycle was double the weight of many of the bikes, but I didn't mind. I just recall this adrenalin rush and thinking 'I'm back in the game'. Johnno and I'd had experiences together kayaking but this was different. This was the sport I was training for when I had my accident.

When I compete in triathlons against able-bodied athletes my hand-cycle leg is always slower than their bike legs. This day lots of the competitors were finishing off the run leg as I was heading out to start it in my wheelchair. I was really pushing it, trying to stay focused on what I needed to do, but finding enough extra to say 'G'day' to a few of the guys I'd met previously. The course had some steep hills and people were saying, 'Can I give you a push?' They were trying to be supportive but I wanted to complete the event by myself. 'No thanks, I'm okay.' I was inching up some of those steep hills but eventually I made it to the finish line as many of the other competitors were preparing to depart.

Even though we had separated Michelle was there, as was Marion, and our dog, a German shepherd called Sasha. Johnno was waiting for me, of course, and people were clapping and cheering. Some kids on the side of the course wore puzzled expressions on their faces as they tried to work out what was happening and why a guy in a wheelchair was in the race. A photograph someone took of those kids looking at me is one of my most treasured possessions. I looked exhausted but I felt different about myself—and I think that shows. Life changed for me that day. For the first time since being hit by the truck I connected back into competitive sport. I crossed the finish line and was welcomed into the bosom of the triathlon family. I was back!

CHAPTER SEVEN

SEEKING THE TRUTH

'I have learnt the ability to "do" through John.
Everything can be done with the right approach
and discipline and the right people around you'
—DAVID KNIGHT, BEST MATE

Ｎone of my family or friends ever mentioned the truck driver whose vehicle hit me on that fateful day. I don't know if they were apprehensive about my reaction or whether they felt bringing it up would serve no useful purpose. But the conversation never took place. I too pushed him to the back of my mind. There wasn't a time when I stopped and reflected on what happened in the cabin of that truck in the moments before it hit me and immediately afterwards. What could I do about it? I couldn't turn back the clock, so for the next two decades I focused on moving forward.

Two acquaintances, however, did raise it. One of the police officers who attended the scene of the accident did so indirectly a couple of years later, sending me a copy of the police report, which included the truck driver's name and address. I spoke to this officer a few times over the years and when I asked him why he'd done it he just said, 'I thought you might want it.' I kept the report for a few years but eventually threw it away as part of a clean-up of old personal documents. I did glance at the name, but it didn't stick in my memory. I was trying to forget, not remember, and I discarded the report along with all the other paperwork that tied me to that day.

The other person who raised the truck driver was a guy I used to play football against who belonged to a bikie gang. It was a year or so after the accident. We worked out at the same gym and he approached me one day while I was bench-pressing weights and said, 'I like you, Maclean—do you know who did this to you?' I said, 'Yes.' His next words charged the air like static electricity: 'I can take care of it for you if you want.' I didn't ask what he meant and I wasn't tempted to find out. 'That would just make it worse for both of us,' I said. 'Thanks, but no thanks.'

I had no intention of trying to find the truck driver before I started working on this book. But as I continued the road trip through my life, it dawned on me he was the last dark spot in my past that I had not confronted head on. I had gone back to the scene of the accident, to the spinal unit at RNS, to Governor Phillip Special Hospital, to the family home in Tregear, to the state records department to access my birth mother Avril's psychiatric report, to her gravesite at Pinegrove Cemetery in Minchinbury just off the Great Western Highway, and to The Gap at Watson's Bay where she had jumped to her death.

If my life were to come full circle, maybe that included meeting the truck driver?

When I first thought about a face-to-face encounter, even I was surprised at my reaction. The mere thought of it was like touching a raw nerve. I don't like negativity, and the potential for conflict that such a meeting could engender made me uneasy. After all these years it remained an issue, a delicate one locked deep in my mind.

Maybe we do bury things that matter. Maybe we hide away the unpleasant episodes of our life because they are more painful than we care to let on. Maybe it was time I faced up to this one. But was the truck driver still alive? Could he be found after all this time when I didn't even remember his name or address? Did he want to be found? And if he was found, would he want to talk to me or be prepared to meet?

These questions were unresolved in my mind when I entered the fifth floor of the NSW Supreme Court and opened the faded manila folder that contained the transcripts of my court case. This was the last stop on my road trip. I had come here to see if there were any surprises in the hundreds of pages of evidence that were given, including testimonies from my dad, Michelle, Professor John Yeo, my football coach at Warragamba, Mark O'Reilly, my physical education teacher at Dunheved High School, David Linback, and even a representative from the Metropolitan Fire Brigade, who was there to verify I had passed the fire brigade entrance exam and would have been offered a position. (I sat the exam before going to court as part of my case about loss of future earnings.)

It struck me this day how life is a series of sliding doors: one shuts as another opens.

As I opened the folder, there, typed in black and clearly legible on the introductory page was the truck driver's name and address. I don't know why it is, but when something is written down it seems more real. Seeing his name staring out from the page somehow turned him into a living, breathing human being.

At that moment I decided to try to find him. I harboured no ill will. All I wanted was the truth and, if I were honest with myself, a belated apology. I also thought that I might be able to help him. Maybe the accident had haunted him all these years and meeting me might provide closure. Maybe he too was waiting to move on with his life.

It dawned on me that what I was contemplating doing was forgiving him. I had forgiven Avril and that had helped me overcome the abandonment issues I had carried since childhood. Maybe forgiving the truck driver would be just as cathartic.

If I could find him and talk to him, I would also be creating another memory of that day that would be easier to carry around inside my head. I had no idea what would happen if we met, what his explanation would be, what he would say. I couldn't control that, and that was quite confronting for me. But I have never shied away from a challenge and I have never hidden from fear—at least not consciously—and suddenly this seemed like a good idea. 'Yes, I have met the truck driver,' I would be able to say. 'We're never going to be friends, but the accident affected his life too.'

This was all swirling through my head as I kept on reading. Then I was brought back to reality with a thud. There, jumping out at me from the pages of the transcript, was another buried incident from the past. Michelle had been pregnant at the time of the court case and while it was early days—the first trimester—there was a due date, January 1992. Her pregnancy, like the truck driver, I had buried deep in my mind, and seeing the fact of it written down took me completely off guard. Suddenly I felt humbled. So much had happened since then it seemed another lifetime ago.

'When your baby is born you have said you are going to go back to work as soon as possible after that, is that the position?' the QC asked Michelle. 'Yes,' she responded. 'How soon after the birth of your child are you anticipating that would be?' 'Well, it really depends on my work, whether I can get maternity leave. I haven't really spoken to them yet,' she said. 'What is the range of time that you had in your mind depending on your work?' 'About a month or two. I really haven't sat down and thought about it.' 'What are you going to do with this one- or two-month-old baby when you go back to work?' 'My mum would have to look after it.' 'Is that your plan or not, leaving it with your mother or not?' 'Or John, one of the two,' Michelle said. 'John would be quite capable as far as you perceive it now of looking after the baby, would he?' 'Yes.'

I could be the father of a seventeen-year-old son or daughter. I closed the file and left the building. I rang Michelle immediately and apologised for not being as sympathetic or understanding as I should have been at the time. We talked about how she had come home from work one day and felt ill and asked me to drive her to the hospital, where she miscarried not long afterward. I don't know that I ever grieved the loss of that baby, certainly not like Michelle did. And I know I wasn't as present in the moment as I should have been. Michelle has been such an important person in my life and I will always love her, even though we went in separate directions.

My visit to the Supreme Court was important because it made me revisit two events that I had long kept hidden from myself. It struck me this day how life is a series of sliding doors: one shuts as another opens.

I was pleased I had been able to talk to Michelle about the child we had lost. I needed to apologise from a vantage point that gave me a sense of perspective and understanding that I didn't have at the time. And I was pleased I'd seen the truck driver's name and address. I didn't know whether we would ever meet, even whether he was still alive, but I was determined to try. Talking to him would take away the power of not knowing what happened on that freeway twenty years ago, and that would be worthwhile.

I have faced many hard realities in my life, and as I grow older I believe one of my strengths is that I have never hidden from fear. I don't want to look back on my life in another twenty years and have any regrets about things I haven't faced up to.

CHAPTER EIGHT

PERSISTENCE

*'He has achieved extraordinary things and has
overcome the most dire of circumstances yet he
is just a humble bloke'*

—TRENT TAYLOR,
JOHN MACLEAN FOUNDATION

I don't have to be told that life can turn on a pin. One minute I was cycling down a freeway without a care in the world, the next I was fighting for my life and coming to terms with injuries so severe they put me in a wheelchair. Of course I asked myself the obvious question, 'Why me?' I've had a lot of time to think about that over the years. Was the accident destiny or fate or just plain bad luck?

I didn't arrive at my conclusion easily or quickly. I don't mind admitting that for a long time I struggled to find any purpose in all that pain and suffering.

But the events of 1995 changed all that. I started believing that things in life are meant to be. I wouldn't put my hand up to be hit by a truck again. No way. But my life post-accident has served a purpose and I think that purpose is to give hope to people that anyone can overcome adversity and go on to do extraordinary things.

I am rushing ahead of myself though. Before I get to 1995 it is important to say something more about what happened after the Nepean Triathlon.

Rather than feel content in the knowledge that I had achieved what I set out to do before the accident, the triumph I felt in finishing that triathlon only inspired me to go further. The fire in my belly that had been feeding my sporting ambition was now a raging inferno. I began looking for new challenges, new ways to prove I was the equal of able-bodied athletes and deserved to be treated with the same respect. I had enjoyed the first sweet taste of success and was hooked. I also started feeling better about myself.

> But my life post-accident has served a purpose and I think that purpose is to give hope to people that anyone can overcome adversity and go on to do extraordinary things.

With Johnno at my side I entered the Sri Chinmoy in early 1995, a well-known Canberra triathlon popular with competitors from all over the country. The event comprises a 2.2-kilometre swim, an 80-kilometre cycle and a 20-kilometre run. Learning from my experience in the Nepean Triathlon I sought out a proper racing wheelchair, rather than the day chair I used for the Nepean Triathlon. Johnno and I set off to do the event together. All was going well until I realised I was labouring during the cycle leg more than I should have been. It took quite a few more kilometres to realise a strap was holding the brake in place and hadn't been released properly before I set off.

I finished the event and immediately started looking for another challenge. My goals had a greater intensity about them now. Looking back, I'm sure they helped distract me from the sobering fact that I was in a wheelchair. Someone once asked me, 'What do you think of when you are awake at night in the dark? What goes through your mind?' The truth is I have always trained so hard that the minute my head hits the pillow I am completely out to it. Rarely do I lie awake pondering life's great mysteries. Is training, then, a way to avoid facing midnight anxiety attacks? I can't say yes, because that is not the truth. I know, however, that sport, especially after the accident, gave me a reason to get up in the morning and made me so tired it put me to sleep at night, and that is a healthy way to live.

Not long after getting back from Canberra I was at Marion and Tony's place watching *Wide World of Sports* on the Nine Network when I saw a segment on the infamous Hawaii Ironman. Better known overseas, especially in the United States where it has cult-like status, this event is to triathletes what the World Cup is to football, the World Series to baseball, the Tour de France to cycling. It is *the* world championships. Tens of thousands of triathletes seek entry each year, but only about 1500 succeed in making it to the starting line at Kona on the 'Big Island', the desolate volcanic island actually called Hawaii. Athletes must either win one of the qualifying events held around the world or jag a spot through the lottery that the organisers run each year. Once there, they must battle the harsh climatic conditions and even harsher terrain in what has become known as the world's toughest endurance event.

An ironman comprises a 3.8-kilometre swim, 180-kilometre cycle and a full 42.2-kilometre marathon. The Hawaii Ironman has been made world famous because of television coverage documenting the incredible feats of human endeavour that are demonstrated each year as athletes, young and old, men and women, strive to finish what they started. One of the most enduring images was of Julie Moss, who in 1982 was leading the women with only 30 metres to go. Exhausted and unable to stand, she crawled to the finish line, only to be pipped at the post. After swimming, cycling and running 226 kilometres she lost the race in the last 15 metres, but was hailed a hero for having made it to the line. Such is the nature of this event, and the way it pits mind against body under such extreme conditions, that the heroes are not always the winners.

Like any triathlete I knew about the race but what transfixed me this day was the story of American Jon Franks, who in 1994 became the first wheelchair athlete to take part in the event. He didn't finish the gruelling course, but his inclusion was a first as organisers sought to establish whether a wheelchair category should be added. In an interview afterward Franks indicated he would be back to try again in 1995. It was like a light bulb went on in my head. 'How cool is this? How special is that guy?' I thought. 'This is what I want to do. I want to go to Hawaii.'

What I didn't know at the time was the intense politics surrounding the inclusion of a wheelchair athlete in the event. Apparently Franks was initially denied entry as it was felt that wheelchair athletes posed safety issues to other competitors and problems for the many volunteers who manned the course.

How would they get Franks in and out of the water? How could they keep an eye on him during the 3.8-kilometre swim? Was that even a problem? What were his medical requirements and what sort of extra training would the volunteers need?

Nonetheless, the World Triathlon Corporation was committed to widening the appeal of the event and knew that for a wheelchair athlete to finish the course would be one of those great human-interest stories that would gain worldwide press coverage and open another door to challenged athletes everywhere. There was a lot at stake. When Franks dropped out of the race in 1994 the nay-sayers grew more vocal. No one at that stage knew if a wheelchair athlete could complete the distance. The last thing the WTC wanted was for a wheelchair athlete to try again and fail. That would send entirely the wrong message.

I was blissfully unaware of all this, of course. It was probably just as well. I wanted to be the first wheelchair athlete to finish the Hawaii Ironman and to make the cut-off times. If I could achieve those feats no one could ever say I wasn't equal, least of all me.

I had set the bar high but wasn't about to dip my toe in the water until I had established I was truly competitive. Could I beat Franks? Were my times even in the ballpark? I found out that he had competed in the Surfer's Paradise International Triathlon—the SPIT—the previous year and thought, 'This is it. That's where I'm off to.' Work and family commitments prevented Johnno from coming with me so another of my mates, David Wells, who's a paramedic, agreed to make the trip to Queensland with me. It was now early 1995.

I completed the course about 45 minutes ahead of Franks' time. Only one word came to mind. 'Aloha,' I told myself.

I contacted the race director for the Hawaii Ironman, Shaaron Ackles, straightaway. She wrote back explaining that to qualify I needed to race off against Franks in the Gulf Coast Triathlon in Panama City, Florida. As the wheelchair section of the Hawaii Ironman was technically still a demonstration event, only one of us could compete. The Gulf Coast Triathlon is held in May, and while it is only a half-Ironman in terms of the distance covered it would give them an idea of my bona fides.

I arrived in Florida with David as my support crew and was keen to meet Franks. It was an odd feeling being in competition with someone again and I was determined to pay my dues and be respectful. 'I saw you on the television,' I said to him. 'I wanted to meet you and tell you how inspired I was by your efforts.' Franks didn't respond to flattery and immediately started grilling me about my times for the swim and the cycle legs. He did backstroke instead of freestyle and must have been keen to compare. 'My times are going to be nowhere near yours,' I told him. I didn't want to give anything away but I thought, 'I'm going to flog you.'

I don't know why it is that people feel that all physically challenged people must get on and like each other, just as I imagine they believe all Aborigines or Pacific Islanders must gel with each other. Franks and I were in competition for a spot in the biggest event in our lives and neither of us was going to back down or roll over. That doesn't mean I am not grateful for the trailblazing he did on behalf of challenged athletes. I am. He was the person who opened the event to us all—but now I had to beat him, pure and simple.

The event had different categories of competitors, including one for challenged athletes that included amputees and the visually impaired. Franks and I were the only wheelchair athletes. Our category went out first.

To my delight I won the swim leg. Although I emerged from the water puffing and panting I was clearly in the lead. David was there waiting for me in the water and after I swam onto his back he started carrying me across the sand to the transition area for the cycle leg. People were clapping and cheering us. Unfortunately David lost his footing in the sand and fell flat on his face with me sprawled out on top of him. 'What are you doing?' I said. 'Get up, you big palooka!'

David struggled to his feet, covered in sand, picked me up and we made our way to my wheelchair where I stripped off the wetsuit and transferred to the hand-cycle as quickly as I could. Because the race had a staggered start I was leading all the other competitors, including the professionals, and I took off on the second leg with a police escort and the lead car, and a film crew trailing me. It wasn't too long before the professional athletes were out of the water, on their bikes and flying past me. I lost my entourage as they took off after the leaders, but I had my moment in the sun.

I'd burned Franks off in the swim leg, but he had much better, more aerodynamic road-racing equipment than mine. I just wanted to stay ahead of him. It was like I was running scared—you know that feeling you get as a kid when you're being chased and don't want anyone to catch up? I was unsure how much of a lead I had when David appeared behind me in a four-wheel-drive with the swimming director, who had befriended us earlier in the week. 'You're well ahead,' David shouted. 'He's got no chance of catching you, keep going, you're on fire.'

I crossed the finish line ecstatic that I had beaten Franks and had qualified for the Hawaii Ironman. I found out later that he had withdrawn from the race after the cycle leg, but he'd lodged a protest anyway, claiming I was swimming off the boat in the swim. Challenged athletes were permitted to have a boat accompany them during the swim leg and David had used a surf ski because he was a trained lifesaver and experienced in using it. I couldn't imagine how there could be any advantage, and the race officials quickly agreed. Franks' protest was dismissed.

The Gulf Coast Triathlon was important because it was my passport to Hawaii, but I made a couple of connections while I was in Panama City that proved just as valuable, although for completely different reasons. I'd met a guy called Dr Patrick Connor at dinner one night before the event; he became something of a White Knight for me when I needed financial support later that year. He was an emergency department doctor at a busy Chicago hospital, and we struck up an instant friendship. At the end of the night he said, 'I want to offer you some sponsorship.' I said, 'I don't need anything, thank you.' Not to be dissuaded, he slipped a card into my hand and told me, 'If you ever need me, give me a call.'

The other connection was with family. My dad was married to Margaret before he married Avril, and had three children with her, Don, Morag and Kenny. The night before the Gulf Coast Triathlon I received an unexpected late-night call from Don, who lived in Toronto. Dad had recently visited Don briefly, en route to Scotland, and told him about my attempt to qualify for the Hawaii Ironman. I had met Don once before when he visited Australia in 1983, but we hadn't really bonded at the time, mainly because of the age difference. Now he was saying, 'If you qualify I'll be there for you in Hawaii.' I was stunned. 'Would you honestly come to Hawaii?' I asked. 'Just qualify and I'll be there.' Don was a sports nut and my dream of competing in one of the most gruelling races in the world caught his imagination. 'I can't explain why,' he told me years later. 'You were trying to prove yourself and I thought I should be there. There was no other reason.' I phoned him after I qualified and said, 'We're going to Hawaii.' Don laughed and said, 'Let me see what I can do for you.'

I flew home to Australia feeling on top of the world. There was some media interest in the fact I'd qualified and *Wide World of Sports* filmed a segment on my training regime. It was winter in Sydney and I couldn't help thinking how much better off I'd be back in Florida, where the heat would help me acclimatise to what I would face in Hawaii in October. Don had been able to organise a return ticket to Hawaii through Canadian Airlines, which still flew out of Sydney at that stage, and I asked him to see if they might add Florida to the route, as I had been offered a place there to stay and train. Canadian Airlines agreed and I left Australia with all my gear and plenty of hugs and kisses from friends and family.

Not long after arriving in Florida I was measured up for a new racing wheelchair which I thought would help improve my performance. When I went to collect it the guy asked for payment on the spot, about US$3000. This put me in a real hole. I didn't have anywhere near that amount available on my credit card—I'd assumed I'd be able to pay it off. Luckily I remembered Patrick Connor's offer, and picked up the phone and called him. 'Pat, I'm a bit stuck,' I said, and explained my dilemma. 'Put the guy on the phone,' he said, and proceeded to sort things out with his credit card. 'Good luck, John,' he said, when I took back the phone and thanked him. 'I'll talk to you soon.'

I said earlier that the events of 1995 changed my life. While the Hawaii Ironman was my focus, it wasn't only the race that was important. Everything leading up to it—the fantastic contacts I made, the incredible acts of generosity my involvement evoked, the way the whole thing brought me back to life in a way that I never thought possible—made me realise this was what I had been chasing since the accident.

I didn't want to be in a wheelchair, but suddenly the wheelchair was helping to open doors for me that included world travel and the recognition for sporting ability that I had dreamed of as a boy. It also gave me a way to give back to others—kids in wheelchairs mainly—because after I competed in that event I felt I could look them in the eye and say, 'Anything is possible. If I can do it, so can you.'

A couple of weeks before the Hawaii Ironman I went to stay in Honolulu so I could train around the island of Oahu before the big event. My excitement was building. I was fit, no doubt about it, but I really wasn't well prepared. I had no idea what I was facing or attempting to accomplish. Sure, I had bravado and confidence—but I completely underestimated the battle of mind over body that would have to take place if I were even to finish the course, let alone make the cut-off times. My preparation in Florida had acclimatised me to humid conditions, but I had been training on a flat course, there and now on Oahu. The island of Hawaii, however, is infamous for its heart-breaking hills, and the hot winds that blow so fiercely across the rocky black lava fields—they not only knock the breath from your body but the spirit from your soul.

I had assembled a big team of supporters who flew in about a week beforehand to cheer me on. Johnno—who had married Gail by this stage and had a young son—was flown over by

Canadian Airlines as my coach, organised by Don. David Wells and his wife at the time, Jodie, were there, as were David's mother Anne, my neighbour Peter Wood, and paddling friend Louis McLachlan. My family was present, too. Marion, who had been writing letters to companies on my behalf seeking sponsorship, made the trip, as did Don from Canada.

I didn't know it at the time, but it was seen as a make-or-break year for wheelchair athletes in the event. More than anything else organisers didn't want to keep failing. The President of WTC at the time, Lew Friedland, who has become a good friend, told me some years later they were looking for the athlete who could break the barrier. 'Had you gone only halfway then maybe we would have gone, "Well you know, we have done this twice now, this really is impossible." We might have told the next wheelchair athlete that called us up, "No thanks. We did it. We tried."'

When we got to Kona I was caught up in the atmosphere and energy that seemed to have infused everyone's mood. Among the crowd were some of the best endurance athletes in the world and suddenly I was one of them. They were accepting me into that family and it felt fantastic.

The morning of the race dawned and I woke before the alarm, around 5 am, filled with nervous energy and a good dose of apprehension. I inserted a catheter so that I didn't need to worry about toilet stops, which are problematic when you are a wheelchair athlete. I dressed in a black wetsuit, which I rolled down to the waist, and a singlet. The organisers had agreed to let me wear a wetsuit—the only concession they made—which would help me keep buoyant in the water to compensate for the fact I couldn't use my legs. My support team soon turned up, and I felt grateful they were all there, cheering me on and willing me to do well. I felt their good wishes would sustain me when the going got tough. News crews from the US television network NBC and Australia's Nine Network also turned up. They were following me for the day, anticipating that my progress—or lack thereof—might be the human-interest story they were always looking out for. Would I be the first wheelchair athlete to finish the course and make the cut-off times? If I did, it would be history in the making and make great footage for the networks.

The race was scheduled to start at 7 am, so I left with enough time to register and have my race number—00—drawn on my arm, and to check my gear one last time.

To say it was a hectic scene at Digme Beach, where the race officially starts, would be a massive understatement. With 1500 athletes herded into such a small area, all with large amounts of adrenalin coursing through their veins, plus thousands of excited friends, family members and spectators lining the foreshore and every other vantage point, and hordes of media people with cameras hanging out of helicopters in the skies overhead, it was nothing short of organised chaos. I looked at the scene unfolding in front of me and took a long, deep breath. This was it. Whether I was prepared or not, the race of my life was about to start and it was time to switch on. I blocked everything else out and told my support crew, 'I'm ready. Let's go.'

One of the other competitors saw me and yelled out, 'Hey, this guy's got a wetsuit on.' Before I could muster a reply, Gordon Bell, a fellow competitor, who coincidentally went to the same high school I did and also belonged to the Nepean Triathlon Club, barked back, 'He's a wheelchair athlete, you dickhead.' The heckler was stopped in his tracks and I felt more supported in that moment on that sporting arena than I had at any time other in my career.

At the start of the race the professionals get a ten-yard buffer, and when the cannon goes off everyone starts swimming like there's no tomorrow. I went out hard. Not surprisingly, so did everyone else. Competitors were swimming over the top of me and anyone else in their way. It's not unusual to suffer a broken nose in that churning mix of arms and legs and it was easy to see why. They didn't care if I was a wheelchair athlete or not, which I respected, because this was the world championship. I was gasping for air and swallowing a lot of salt water before moving a little to the side of the course to get out of their way. It was a smart tactic because I went from feeling spent to finding an easy rhythm. I am a strong swimmer and once I found my stroke and concentrated on being as efficient as possible, I moved quickly through the water.

I recorded a good time for the swim, about an hour and seven minutes, and when I approached the shore at the finish of the leg, Johnno and David were there to meet me and carry me out of the water. They put me under the shower to wash the salt off the wetsuit and out of my hair and sat me in the wheelchair, where I stripped down to my racing suit, put on helmet, gloves, sunglasses and shoes, then transferred to my hand-cycle. David put some Vaseline under my arms to prevent chafing and on the back of my neck too—which turned out to be not such a good idea because it contributed to my severe sunburn later on—and with a pat on the back from Johnno I was off again, feeling confident and relatively relaxed.

Apart from finishing the race, there is nothing better in a triathlon than starting well and being in front of a lot of the other competitors early on, especially for wheelchair athletes, who get overtaken in the cycle leg because a hand-cycle is slower than a racing bike, primarily because it is powered by the arms, not the legs. We normally make up ground again in the run, because we use a racing wheelchair, but the cycle leg is where it's easy to lose heart and resolve as other competitors fly past. At this point, however, I was feeling none of that. I had easily made the cut-off time in the swim and had 9 hours and 20 minutes to hand-cycle 180 kilometres.

The first hill at the start of the cycle leg was a steep one. Thousands of spectators had jagged their spots along the road early and had written messages to loved ones like, 'Reg you can do it. We are with you.' Everyone was clapping and cheering and urging me on, and I was caught up in the whole atmosphere. After scaling the hill the course turned onto Queen Kaahumanu Highway—better known as the Queen K—a long, long stretch of road with undulating hills that loomed ominously before me. Every 10 kilometres there was an aid station, staffed by volunteers handing out Gatorade and water and bananas and glucose—everything you needed. They were very encouraging, yelling out, 'Come on mate,' and I was still thinking, 'This is fantastic.'

But as the morning wore on, the conditions that had seemed quite welcoming and tame in the beginning suddenly became my enemy. The Queen K is set in the middle of a vast tract of black volcanic rock that absorbs the sun's rays and then acts like a giant natural heater, spewing the warmth back up into the atmosphere. I felt like I was in an oven, baking, which wasn't helped by the fact I was sitting so low to the bitumen. I could feel the heat radiating off the road and wondered at one stage if I wouldn't start melting. Not only that, but the wind, which is notorious in this part of the world, suddenly picked up strength and went from a gentle breeze flirting with the back of my hair to a full-on headwind, which halved my speed and forced me to cycle in the lowest gear. My entire upper body was cramping, but I was loath to stop in case both biceps and triceps went into spasm. I was hurting, to say the least.

It took me five hours to reach the halfway point—then I had to turn around and do it all again in reverse. What I wasn't aware of until then was that the trade winds take a 180-degree shift in the early afternoon. I had been banking on the fact that the wind would be behind me once I turned around, but it was hitting me head-on again. It was a clear case of double jeopardy. I felt my spirits sink as the enormity of the job at hand became clear.

This is a race that disadvantages any athlete who is on the course for a long time. If you are a professional and can cycle fast, then you ride with the wind. But if you are a hand-cyclist and you are taking a very long time, you get the headwind on the way out and on the way back. That's why this event tests athletes so much and why finishing the course becomes the ultimate goal. I understood that now, just as I appreciated how ill prepared I was. Sure, I was unlucky that the wind gusts were reaching a speed of 100 kilometres an hour, the worst such conditions in more than ten years, but I had not realised how much of a mind game it would become. I was being tested at every level and at that stage, I don't mind admitting, I was faltering.

My goal was never to just finish the course. I desperately wanted to make the cut-off times to prove to everybody, but most of all to myself, that I was the equal of any athlete out there. But as the sun started sinking over the horizon, throwing up a brilliant red glow, I couldn't help but think, 'I'm not going to make it. After all of this, I'm going to be disqualified.' They say people find out who they really are on the Queen K. When mind and body are locked in a knockout battle to just keeping going, that is when your true character is revealed. I felt stripped bare and more exposed than I had the time I first saw my wasted body in the hospital mirror.

> Johnno effectively ripped open my chest and squeezed my heart. He made it impossible for me to give up.

The cut-off time for the cycle leg is 5.30 pm. That's when the sun goes down in Hawaii at that time of year, and organisers don't want anyone riding a bike in the dark. Safety is the main reason, because they are responsible for everyone on the course. When it hits 5.30 and you haven't made it to the transition area for the run leg, you are meant to move to the side of the course and that's it. It's over for you. I didn't know it at the time but when it became clear I wasn't going to make it by 5.30, Don started negotiating with the race officials to allow me to continue anyway, arguing that we would provide our own light for safety and our own water and nutritional needs, given a number of the aid stations on the cycle course would be closing. Everyone knew I could do the run leg faster than many of the athletes, because I was quicker in my wheelchair than they were on their legs, but would they let me try? Would they make an exception? And would I agree to it once my dream of making the cut-off times was extinguished?

I had seen Johnno, Don and David on the course during the day, waving Australian flags and urging me on. Don had organised a vehicle and mobile phone to track my progress and initially their presence at various points had a positive impact. It spurred me on. But as conditions took their toll and I didn't make various checkpoints as early as they hoped, they knew I was in trouble. My body was screaming in pain and my mind starting doubting whether this was whole ironman thing was a good idea to start with. I sank lower in the hand-cycle, shoulders hunched, like all the air had been sucked from my body. People who know me well know this is a bad sign. Johnno knew it, just as he knew exactly where on the course I would be feeling it most, where I would be mostly likely to give up.

Once the organisers agreed to let me continue, Johnno ran across a golf course to find me. I had about a kilometre to go and had just reached the base of the last big hill before the transition area. I had made a decision. If I could just make it to the top of the hill I could roll down the other side and finish the cycle leg—and that would be the end of it. I'd given it a good shake. Without doubt it was the hardest day of my life from a sporting perspective and I didn't think anyone could begrudge my withdrawing after doing my best. Johnno could see the pain in my eyes and my hunched position. He said nothing for a while, just walked along beside me. Then he articulated what I knew in my heart already: 'Mate, you've been disqualified. But they're going to let you finish.' 'Johnno, I'm gone,' I said. 'I've got nothing left. I'm not going on.'

I mentioned earlier that I believe things happen for a reason. There were lots of examples that day that proved to me that is absolutely true. It wasn't coincidental that Johnno found me when he did. If we hadn't talked at exactly that moment, I would have called it quits. And if I had given up, there is no doubt my life would have turned out differently. I would have moved in another direction, I'm sure. But my dream of being a professional athlete would have been shattered and my desire to prove I was the equal of any man would have suffered a major setback. I'm not saying my life would have been over but, just like the accident robbed me of the use of my legs, I think failure at that point would have required years of rehabilitation.

But Johnno, tears welling in his eyes, spoke to me from the heart. 'John, you've got to go on,' he said. 'It's my son's birthday today and I'm not with him, I'm with you. You can't stop now.' I had never seen Johnno cry before and it stopped me in my tracks. For six years he had been there by my side. He never gave up visiting me in hospital, never threw in the towel in the gym, never stopped believing that I would walk again. He was my Rock of Gibraltar and my best mate and there was no way I was going to disappoint him. I would have rolled over and died before doing that. I have said before that Johnno effectively ripped open my chest and squeezed my heart that day—and he did. But most of all he made it impossible for me to give up, so I kept on going until I reached the top of the hill and made it down the other side to the transition area where David Yates, the president of WTC, was waiting. 'John, you've been disqualified, you missed the cut-off time by forty minutes,' he said. 'But we would like you to continue if you want to.' I thought, 'I'm tired. I'm ready for bed. I'll see you another time.' Then I looked at Johnno and knew there was no discussion to be had. 'I'll go on,' I said, knowing that not only had I never done a full marathon before, I'd never done one on this unrelenting course that claims among its victims the strongest men and women.

... if you never ever give up, life has a way of rewarding you.

There was no need to rush now. My goal was to finish the course, not make the cut-off times, so I had a drink and caught my breath and said to David's mother Anne, 'Did you see the swim?' 'Yes,' she said. 'I was smokin'.' 'Yes, you were smokin',' she replied. The television cameras were rolling and I was trying to keep a cheerful tone in my voice when all the time I was thinking, 'I'm gone.' Peter Wood, David and Johnno all followed me out on the beginning of the run leg, ostensibly to show me the way, but underneath they knew I faced a near-vertical climb up that first hill. I was about a third of the way up when the front wheel of my three-wheel racing chair started lifting off the road. 'Just how much more difficult can this get?' I thought. David suggested, 'Turn your wheelchair around and take your gloves off and pull up on the spokes.' He meant go up backwards, which is what I did, and it worked. It was slow going as I inched my way up the hill. But at least I was making progress. The cameras were still rolling and while I wasn't aware of it at this stage, that bit of footage would go on to become synonymous with the event, typifying the uphill struggle many athletes face just finishing the course.

I didn't know whether to hug David or curse him. Had he not said anything it would have been all over—I don't think

I would have made it up the hill. But suddenly there I was at the top, turning around again and enjoying the feeling of coasting down the other side. I felt relieved—that is, until another hill loomed in front of me. My pace slowed as I started the climb and when it became too difficult I turned around and went up backwards again. I had nothing left in the tank. I looked at Johnno, who was walking beside me, and in a near-whisper said, 'I've had enough. I'm not enjoying this.' I had slowed to a halt and it suddenly seemed like we were the only two people on earth. He bent down so he could look me squarely in the eye and said, 'The pain won't last forever, but the memories will.'

Where does a guy who normally doesn't say a whole lot come up with two priceless lines on the same day to inspire his best mate? I smiled. How could I not go on?

Then I looked at the cameramen and said, 'Get that on tape, brothers, that was beautiful.' My tank was empty and Johnno had filled it up again. I had started the marathon with him walking slowly beside me. But once I made it over the hill he couldn't run fast enough to keep up. 'It was all my emotion that came spilling out,' Johnno told me later. 'After all that we'd been through together you weren't giving up. That wasn't going to happen unless you were in an ambulance.'

I did struggle for the next couple of kilometres after Johnno spoke those famous words, but it was like a dimmer light was coming back on power. 'You went from Struggle Street to going again because it wasn't the hill that was stopping you, it was your mind,' he said. 'As soon as we talked to each other and talked it all out you took off. I remember going back to the transition area and everyone was so happy. I was so proud. It was the best moment you could imagine as far as a training partner went or a friend. I knew then that I had helped you.'

Johnno had done more than just help me. I didn't know it at the time but he had paved the way for a new life for me. Things would never be the same after 1995. When I talk about that race to business managers and executives in the presentations I do today, I don't dwell on training or preparation or who was the best athlete on the day. I tell them the real lesson to be learned from it was how one person can inspire another, how you can make a difference to someone else's life. I tell them about the importance of friendship and sharing your journey and how I am proof that if you never ever give up, life has a way of rewarding you.

Johnno and I will always be best friends. But we knew we were at a crossroads in our relationship at that time. He had a wife and a young child. The priority he had given me in his life needed to shift to his family. He had helped lift me out of Penguin Place onto the world sporting stage, and for that I can never thank him enough. I think he wanted me to finish what I had started and to make sure I was on my way in this new phase of my life before he stepped aside. It is the greatest gift a person has ever given me.

'The pain won't last forever, but the memories will.'

I would be lying if I said the rest of the race was easy. It wasn't. My arms were shot, and the back of my neck, and my face, were so sunburnt I could feel the skin tightening by the minute. But suddenly finishing the course seemed possible. Two Harley-Davidson motorbikes were travelling behind me, lighting up the road, and people were shouting, 'Here comes the wheelchair guy.' I was like, 'Get out of my way because I'm coming through.' I was gradually picking up other competitors and while it was pain all the way I knew at that point that I would be the first wheelchair athlete in the history of the Hawaii Ironman to finish the race. I hadn't made the cut-off times, but as I made my way onto Alii Drive and the last few hundred metres I purposefully slowed down.

The barricades on the side of the road were crammed with people cheering and clapping and I took my gloves off and tried to soak it all up. I wasn't coming back again—at least, that's what I was thinking at the time. Why would I ever put myself through this much pain again? I took out my Australian flag and started waving it and girls were leaning over the barricades kissing me. Music was blaring out of the loud speakers, one pumped-up song after another, and I was thinking, 'How good is this?'

Johnno was the first person I saw as I crossed the finishing line. I did a wheelie as a salute, which was the easiest thing I'd done all day. It had taken me 14 hours and 52 minutes to complete the course and I think I was in agony for at least ten of those hours. The total race cut-off time was 17 hours, which I had made, but because I missed the cycle cut-off time I didn't get a finisher's medal. Johnno gave me a slap on the back, which was as close as he got to a cuddle with another man, then Marion hugged me so hard she nearly broke my neck, and Don was there with a flower lei.

I was carted off by race officials and taken to the medical centre where I was put on an IV drip, but at that moment I didn't care about the pain in my arms or the severe sunburn or about being dehydrated and exhausted.

Nothing could have wiped the smile from my face.

CHAPTER NINE

CHASING MY DREAMS

*'No human being in a wheelchair has even come
remotely close to the accomplishments he's had.
No one anywhere in the world'*
—LEW FRIEDLAND, FORMER PRESIDENT,
WORLD TRIATHLON CORPORATION

I am not the sort of person who keeps my trophies in glass cabinets. Nor do I frame and hang the photographs taken of me with the sporting legends I have met over the years. In fact, people are often surprised when they first visit me and find no visible memorabilia to attest to the life I have lived. Those few keepsakes I truly value I keep locked away in a cupboard.

That said, after the 1995 Hawaii Ironman I did say to Don, 'Are you sure they're not going to give me a medal?' 'No one has ever done what you've done,' he said. 'This is bigger than a piece of metal.' The answer, of course, was no, they weren't. It did bother me, though, because I had no intention at that point of returning to Hawaii and putting myself through the physical and mental anguish I had just endured.

The medical staff checked me out after the race and Don escorted me back to the hotel room we shared in Kona. It was after midnight by the time we got there. While my exhausted body screamed for rest, my mind was in overdrive. I had been on an emotional roller-coaster for almost eighteen hours and while the ride was over the memory of it was red raw, just like the sunburn on my arms, neck and face. Don drew me a cold bath and I sat in the water with the bathroom door closed, taking a private moment to reflect on what had happened during the day. When I finally crawled between the sheets I can't remember my head hitting the pillow.

I slept more soundly that night than I ever had before. When I woke in the morning I could barely move. My shoulders and upper arms ached so much I wondered if they'd gone into spasm. Even opening the door sent a sharp pain searing through me like a switchblade. We met the others for breakfast and as we walked along the side of the road I said to Johnno, 'Can I grab your hand to get me up the street?' I didn't have enough strength left to push my wheelchair. 'That's not going to happen,' he said indignantly. 'You can hold onto my belt buckle, but you're not going to hold my hand.' Johnno was a magical human being but he never openly expressed his love for another male. That changed over the years as he grew older but his predictable macho reaction that day made me laugh—and even that hurt.

Despite the pain racking my body I was on a high. Everywhere we went people were stopping us in the street and congratulating me on the race. I felt like a celebrity at an A-list event. It was such a change. When I left Australia I was still leery of the looks people gave me. I was self-conscious about being in a wheelchair and second-guessed the questions

I thought people wanted to ask or backed away if I detected the slightest glimmer of pity in their eyes. Now I was lauded for what I had been able to do with my physical challenges and it was a special experience.

Every year on the night after the Hawaii Ironman an awards night is held for competitors who have won their respective race categories. I hadn't intended going but Don eventually persuaded me to. My whole group rocked up and we were stunned at the reception I received. Towards the end of the evening I was lifted onto the stage—to be overwhelmed by the standing ovation they gave me. When I was handed the microphone I felt more butterflies in the pit of my stomach than I did at the start of the event. I admired these athletes so much and here I was, standing before them as a peer. 'You've got to give me a second here, guys, because they're going to kick me off,' I said, trying to quieten the crowd. I thanked everyone who had helped me along the way. In closing I made a joke: 'I don't know why you guys are complaining about your legs. Mine don't hurt at all.' It brought the house down.

I had spent that day with athletes coming up to me and slapping me on the back or squeezing my shoulders in congratulations; in return I'd reach out and squeeze their calf muscles, causing them to flinch or jump just as I did every time someone gave my shoulders a squeeze.

I didn't know it at the time but the event and I were now inextricably linked. The owners of the Hawaii Ironman had always strived to ensure it was not seen as elitist, and by that I respectfully mean not dominated by men and women whose physical prowess defies description. They wanted television viewers everywhere to be inspired by the courage and spirit of the everyday people who were realising their dreams by just finishing the course. These were the people who'd gained entry via the lottery system, and their stories, whether they had to walk, crawl or, in my case, turn a wheelchair around to get up the hills backwards, were used to define the event, when really it defied logic. I was now one of those stories.

Of course I wasn't aware of it then. The extent of the connection would take much longer to sink in. I flew back to Sydney with Johnno a couple of days later. Like the true friend she has always been, Michelle picked me up from the airport and drove me home. It seemed a world away from the experiences we'd just come through, and that's probably because it was. They talk about the 'ironman blues' that a lot of competitors suffer after events such as the one in Hawaii. Athletes train so hard for so long, taking them away from their families and the natural rhythm of ordinary life. When it's over they feel euphoric at having achieved their goals but after a few days there is a massive letdown. They're tired, some of them feel depressed, and many of them feel lost.

I think I went through that. I didn't do much for a long time except sleep, eat and watch movies. It took my body and my mind weeks to find equilibrium and I drifted aimlessly for a while, which is very unlike me.

The next few months ticked by and it wasn't until early 1996, January or February, that I started thinking about Hawaii. At first I quickly dispelled any notion of competing again. But the more I thought of it the more intrigued I became by the idea. I hadn't decided for sure whether I would commit to it until I was at home one night watching *Dead Poet's Society* once again. One of the famous lines of the English professor trying to inspire his students to chase their dreams was 'Gather ye rosebuds while ye may'—and this night it stuck in my mind.

Was that what I should do? I didn't have to be told that life was fragile. The accident on the M4 had made that point very clearly seven years earlier. There was no telling what awaits any of us in the future. Maybe it *was* the right thing to do. Maybe I would regret it if I didn't try again. I wasn't jumping up and down and shouting it out from the rooftops, but that's when I made the decision. Four months after pushing myself to the limit I decided I was going back to Hawaii.

By then my life had changed direction. Companies that hadn't been interested in me before were now at least taking my calls to talk about sponsorship. I had attracted some media attention and was learning fast how the two ran hand in hand. I wasn't offered big bucks, certainly not enough to finance even my modest lifestyle, let alone the cost of equipment and funding my training and travel—that was being bankrolled by the little cash I had left from the insurance settlement and by some part-time work with Spinesafe—but it was a start.

In May 1995 I qualified for the Hawaii Ironman by beating Jon Franks in Panama City, Florida. In 1996 the qualifying event was to be held in July in Santa Rosa, California. Despite having achieved what no other wheelchair athlete had by finishing the course, I received no free ride. I wasn't guaranteed a place at the starting line. Like everyone else, I had to prove my mettle. And I liked it that way.

I flew back to Panama City, because that's where I had some contacts, and began training in earnest. I entered a number of triathlons and Don flew down from Canada to help organise sponsorship and transport. He'd phone the various race directors and give them a pitch; sometimes they'd be keen to have me involved, and pay our accommodation and provide vehicles. Canadian Airlines gave me first-class air travel again, and some other companies like Nike came on board too, helping out with gear. I was broke and living off my wits but I loved every minute of it.

That year Don gave me something else apart from his time and negotiating expertise—the chance to meet the other members of the Canadian side of my family. I had never met Morag or Kenny and thought it was time I did. I entered a few triathlons in Canada and Don once more went cap in hand to Canadian Airlines. I was so grateful they agreed to help.

I landed in Toronto and was met at the airport by Don. Our first family dinner was a memorable night. Morag greeted me with a rather diffident handshake but Kenny gave me a good old bear-hug. I think Morag suffered the most when Dad left. She was seven at the time and waited for years for him to walk in the front door. I don't think she ever forgave him for not coming back. It took a while to break the ice, but by the end of the night, when we said our goodbyes, it was with a hug that seemed to go on forever. Neither of us wanted to be the one who let go first.

I felt blessed having the opportunity to spend several weeks in Canada with my family. I always enjoy their company and have laughed and marvelled with them at how similar we are in certain ways.

Around this time Don approached Subaru about the possibility of providing a vehicle for us while I competed in Canada and later on in Hawaii. I had a lot of gear by now and really needed a van to move it around. Don put together a promotional package that included a video edited on his home VCR of the 1995 Hawaii Ironman and some magazine articles he'd cut out, and took it into Subaru's head office. He wasn't having much luck getting his foot in the door, so he asked the receptionist if she could get someone to just take a look at the video—and he waited. Shortly afterwards, in tears, a female sales representative came out to talk to him. Don eventually got to see the national sales manager, who said, 'This is an awesome story, but he's not Canadian, he's Australian. We really should have a Canadian.' Then he asked Don, 'Can John talk?' 'Oh yeah, no problem,' Don said. (The truth was, apart from my time at Spinesafe talking to kids in schools, I had done little public speaking.) The sales manager offered us a deal—I would address the company's eastern sales conference because the athlete they usually used as their inspirational speaker couldn't attend that year, and in return they would provide a Subaru vehicle for us in Toronto and later on in Hawaii.

It was our first big sponsorship deal apart from Canadian Airlines and the first time I really appreciated the power of my story, at least as far as other people were concerned. I don't think I am any more special than anyone else. But I do think my story strikes a deep emotional chord. Everyone faces adversity at some time in their life. I give them reason to believe they can bounce back and achieve things after misfortune. After the accident all I was trying to do was re-establish my life and become what I always wanted to be—an athlete. In doing this I unintentionally became an example of the truth that anything is possible if you never give up hope and believe unflinchingly in yourself.

I went to the conference, and when they played the video you could have heard a pin drop. The North American sales manager stood and said, 'This is a special day for me. Most

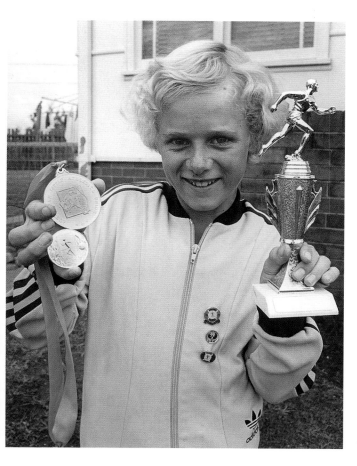

I won my first state
and national title in
little athletics age twelve.

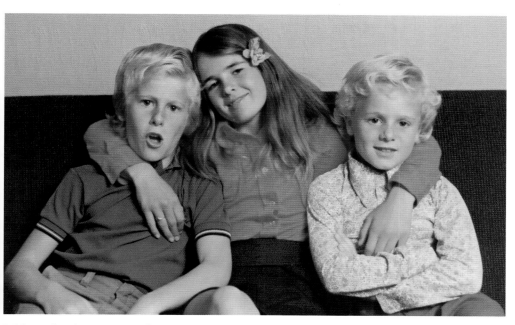

With my brother, Marc, and my sister, Marion. I'm on the right.

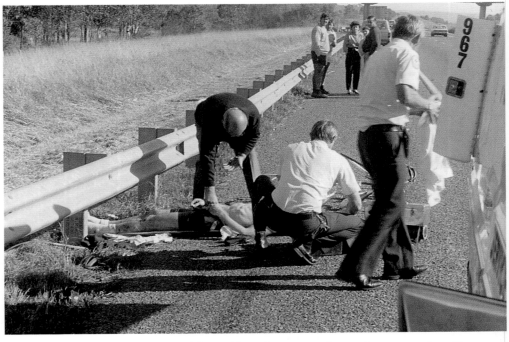

Paramedics treat me at the scene of the accident that was to change the course of my life.

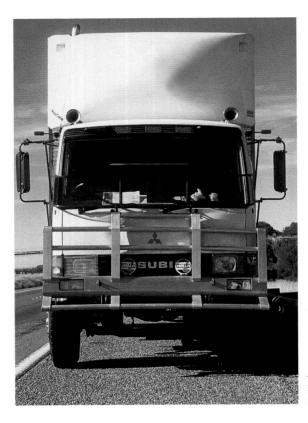

A forensic police photo of the truck that ran into me, taken near the scene of the accident.

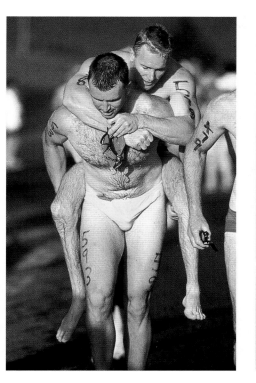

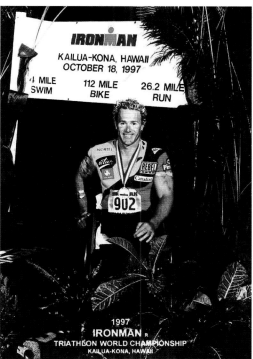

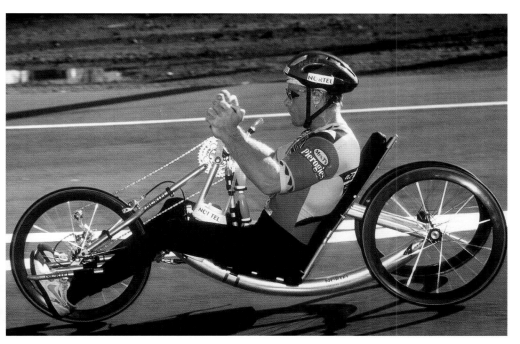

Clockwise from top left: my best mate, Johnno, carries me out of the water after the swim leg of the 1994 Nepean Triathlon; proudly wearing my finisher's medal after the 1997 Hawaii Triathlon; on my handcycle during the cycle leg of the Ironman World Championships in Hawaii 1995. (Photos Delly Carr and World Triathlon Corporation)

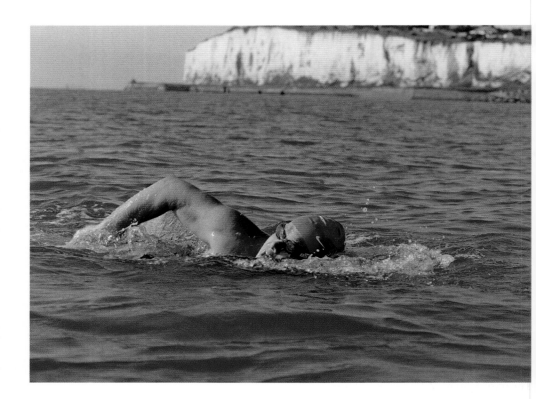

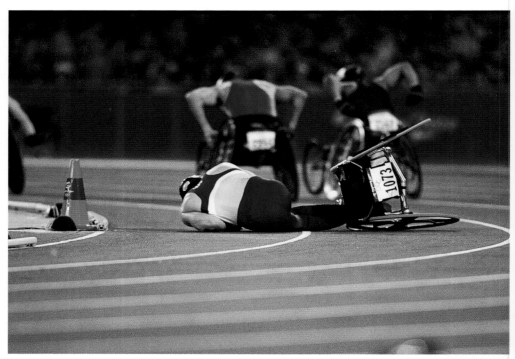

Top: Swimming the English Channel. Bottom: The disastrous crash during the 2000 Sydney Olympic Games (1500 metre demonstration wheelchair race).
(Photos Lisa Saad and Anthony Phelps)

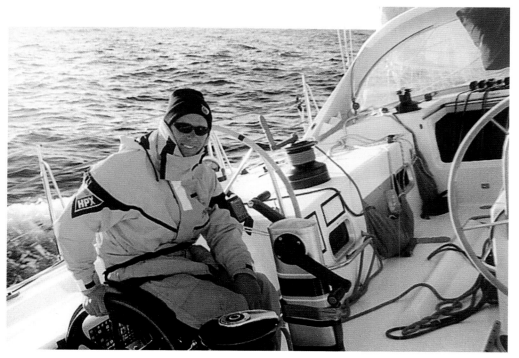

The 2001 Sydney to Hobart Yacht Race.

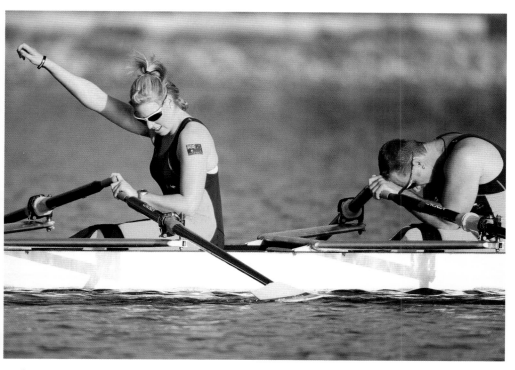

With my rowing partner, Kathryn Ross, at the 2008 Beijing Paralympics. It's the end of the race and my expression says it all. (Photo Getty Images)

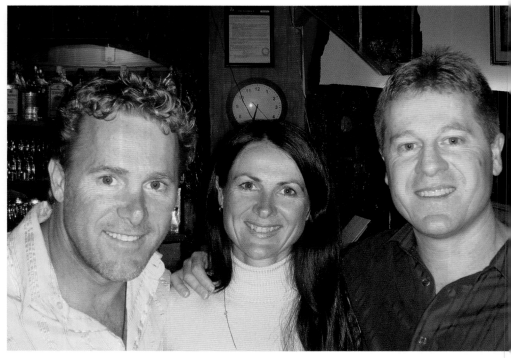

With Marion and Marc, my loving siblings.

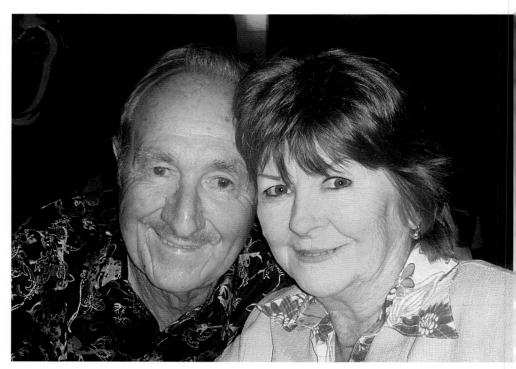

Dad and Mum have always supported me and believed in me.

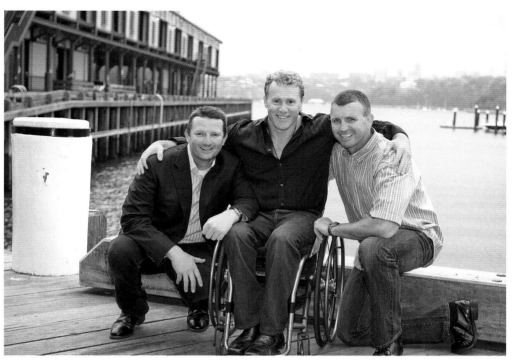

With my best mates David Knight and John Young. (Photo Simon Grimmett)

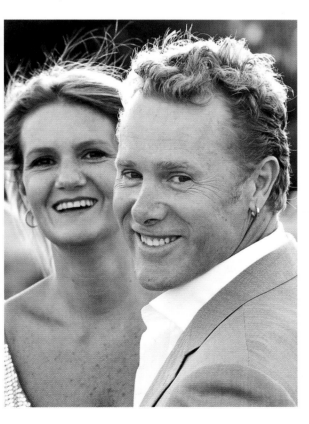

With Amanda on our wedding day, 2009. (Photo Simon Grimmett)

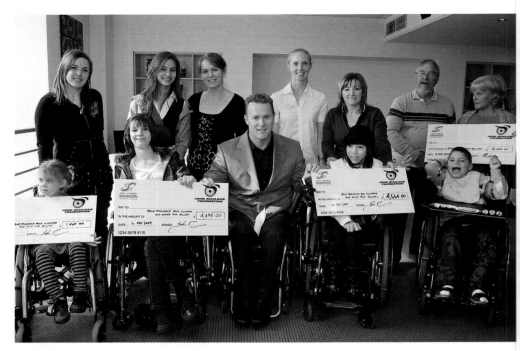

At a presentation in Melbourne where the John Maclean Foundation gave almost $50 000 in funding to assist with the purchases of new wheelchairs, vehicle modifications and remedial aids for young wheelchair users. (Photo Lisa Saad)

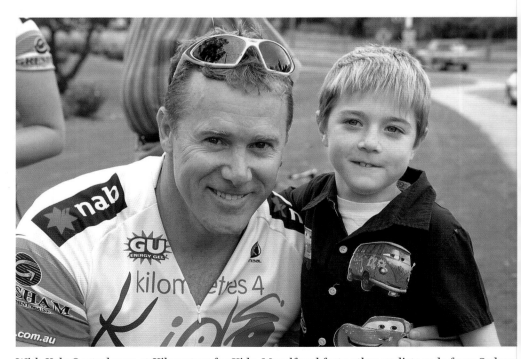

With Kyle Oosterkamp at Kilometres for Kids. Myself and forty other cyclists rode from Sydney to Melbourne to raise funds for the John Maclean Foundation and present kids like Kyle, who suffers from muscular dystrophy, with grants. (Photo Lisa Saad)

of you know that my child is in a wheelchair and I wish she were here today.' Then he introduced me. I gave a short talk about my life and what I was doing now and my plans for the future and received a standing ovation. It was my first time in front of such a crowd, but whenever I speak I do so from the heart, and the people there appreciated that. I also understand that most people have been touched by sadness in their life. If not themselves then they know someone who has been dealt a poor hand. Like the North American sales manager, it might be their own child who is in a wheelchair, or someone else close to them who is suffering an illness, or maybe it's the death of a loved one. Bad things happen to us all at some point in our lives and I think I am living proof it needn't define who we are.

After the conference I returned to Panama City, where I was dating a beautiful woman called Cynthia whom I had met the previous year. I wasn't finding it difficult attracting female attention. I've always found it easy talking to women—my dad has the gift of the gab and I'm sure some of it's rubbed off on me. But I also think there is something non-threatening about a man in a wheelchair that gives women the confidence to strike up a conversation. Once I was comfortable in my own skin and had accepted the wheelchair and my new image, I think other people did too.

It was Cynthia who accompanied me to Santa Rosa for the qualifying event. I was the only wheelchair athlete competing, so all I had to do was complete the course to earn the right to take another crack at Hawaii. The race was a half-Ironman comprising a 1.9-kilometre swim, 90-kilometre cycle and 21.1-kilometre run, all of which went according to plan. I used it as a training run to test my endurance and the capabilities of my new hand-cycle. In 1995 I'd had no trouble making the cut-off times for the swim and marathon. It was the cycle leg that had been my downfall, and I knew if I were to get a medal this year that's where the improvement had to be made. I'd had a new hand-cycle made specifically, which was lighter and more manoeuvrable than the old one, and I hoped this would give me the edge I needed.

After the Santa Rosa race, Cynthia and I returned to Florida and I moved in with her. We were spending a lot of time together anyway so it made sense. She had a big enough place to accommodate all my gear and lived near the beach, which was a great place to finalise my preparation. I had devised my own training regime and was working on improving my strength for hand-cycling, and my endurance. My new equipment gave me confidence that this was my year.

A week before the race I flew out to Hawaii. Little had changed in Kona and not surprisingly I had strong feelings of *déjà vu* as I wheeled around the little fishing village where just twelve months earlier I experienced so much pain. On the one hand it seemed like a lifetime ago but on the other it seemed like yesterday. This time my support crew was much smaller. It included Kylie Nicholson, a masseuse from Penrith who had spent many hours working on my shoulders after the 1995 event. I appreciated the battering my upper body—my shoulders, in particular—took after that first attempt and knew they needed to be treated with the respect they deserved. Cynthia joined me a few days before the race, as did Don. I was attracting quite a bit of media attention and NBC, the American television network, asked if they could film me the day before the race hand-cycling up some of the hills. I agreed, because I thought the exposure would be helpful. Every year

NBC produces a documentary of the event that has, overall, won fourteen Emmy awards and thirty-nine nominations. But it was crazy to be out there expending energy the day before the race, and I regretted it later.

The night before the race I was pretty relaxed, although I couldn't quite shake a slight feeling of unease that had been dogging me since I arrived. I couldn't pinpoint what it was exactly, although some have suggested since it was a premonition. 'Something just doesn't feel right,' I said to Kylie, but then I dismissed it as normal pre-race jitters.

I woke the morning of the race feeling confident but nervous. The hotel we had booked was closer to the course than last year's accommodation so it was a short trip down to the beach to the starting line. Two guys I knew, Tim Twardzik and Ernest Ferrell, carried me into the water and everything was in place. The cannon sounded and I was off again. I was the only wheelchair athlete competing but at this point that was irrelevant. In this event you battle the course and the conditions more than anything else as well as your own body and mind. The advantage I had this year was that I was better prepared and I knew what I was in for. I also knew I could do it.

My swim leg was good. I knew to move to the side of the course to avoid being caught in the swirl of eager competitors and quickly established a rhythm. I beat my time of the previous year by two minutes, and Tim and Ernest were waiting for me. They carried me out of the water, put me through the shower and into my wheelchair where I changed for the cycle leg. It was a seamless transition and before I knew it I was on the road, heading off towards the Queen K and the black rocky lava fields that had made my first attempt a living hell. In 1995 I engaged with the other athletes, yelling out 'G'day', and talking to the television crews along the course. There was none of that this year. I was fitter, my hand-cycle was lighter, I was more aware of my nutritional needs and of staying properly hydrated and I thought, 'This is it. I'm going to make it.'

With only about 50 kilometres to go in the cycle leg, I was hurting, but aware I had to keep my heart rate up to ensure I maintained speed. I was trying to stay focused when I felt the hand-cycle falter underneath me—the right rear tyre had blown. This not only slowed me down, it made it more difficult to manoeuvre. I was 5 kilometres from the next aid station and felt my heart sinking in my chest. 'Why now?' I thought. 'Why here?'

Many people have asked, 'What was the problem? Why didn't you just change it on the spot?' If you can walk, you can change a tyre easily. You get off your bike, crouch down on the side of the road and do it. But when you are a paraplegic, you have to *sit* on the side of the road. While conditions were nowhere near as fierce as the previous year, the bitumen was still too hot to touch. I made the only safe decision I could—to continue on with the flat tyre until I reached the aid station and found an area with some grass where I could sit down and change it. I knew it would cost me precious minutes and possibly jeopardise my chances of success. But what else could I do?

Eventually I made it and found a patch of grass. Athletes must change their own tyres and we all carry the necessary equipment. The volunteers looked on dutifully. No one said anything but I could tell they were mentally computing my chances of making up the lost time. Now I was in desperate trouble against the clock. It was going to be close, very close.

I was telling myself over and over, 'This can still happen, keep going, stay positive.' But as I saw the sun dipping in the sky I started feeling anxious. When I finally wheeled into the transition area, race director Shaaron Ackles was waiting for me with an unmistakable look of disappointment in her eyes. I knew instinctively what was coming: 'John, you have been disqualified. You have missed the cut-off by fifteen minutes. But please go on. There are people waiting for you at the finish line.'

What could I say? More to the point, what could I do? Everything I had done to prepare for this race went through my mind. The early morning training rides in Panama City, where other cyclists would call out to me, 'Hey, superhero!' and I would wave and keep riding; the triathlons I had competed in around Canada and in the USA; and the promises I had made to myself and everyone else in my life that, yes, this year would be the one. I felt like a whipped dog with its tail between its legs. But I looked up into Shaaron's eyes and said the only thing I could under the circumstances, 'I'll go on and finish.'

I transferred to my racing wheelchair and set off to face that first, steep hill. It was one of the hardest things I've had to do. My dream was in tatters but I knew I had to finish, so I mustered all the courage and strength I could find within myself and I kept going. Like the previous year I started picking up other competitors and overtaking them. The 42.2 kilometres went by in a blur. I had gone into the zone, blocking out what happened during the day and what it all meant for me.

I was in pain. No one finishes a Hawaii Ironman without taking their body to the brink. But when I approached the finishing line the scene that awaited me was spectacular. The music was blaring and the spectators were fifteen deep along the barricades, clapping and cheering me and throwing out their hands for a high five. I pulled out the Australian flag again and waved it proudly as I crossed the line. It had taken me 14 hours and 39 minutes, 13 minutes better than in 1995. Even though I was disappointed I would be lying if I said it wasn't a special moment. It was. They gave me a towel and after I wheeled off the course they put a medal around my neck. I was stunned.

> Sometimes you don't get it right the first time. But keep going, keep chasing your dreams because the journey is just as important as the destination.

I made a point of getting an IV drip after the race to rehydrate quickly, and a massage to soothe my aching shoulders and arms. Then I went to my hotel room, had a shower, put on some jeans and a T-shirt and went back to the finishing line to cheer on the other athletes. Lots of competitors do that and that's why there's such a great feeling of camaraderie at the finish. As the last athlete crossed the finish line the guy calling the race on the microphone called me over. 'Ladies and gentlemen, this is John Maclean.'

I felt great until Don confronted me about the medal. 'You've got to give it back,' he said. 'What do you mean, I've got to give it back?' I replied. 'You didn't make the cut-off time and you've got to give it back.' I was crestfallen, but I knew he was right. No matter how much I wanted that medal as a keepsake of the time and effort I had put into this event, it meant nothing if I hadn't earned it. The next morning I rang Shaaron and drove to the office to meet her. 'There's been a mistake,' I said. 'I'm handing the medal back.' She refused to take it, saying, 'If anyone deserves it, John, you do.' She was crying and we had a cuddle. I didn't know what else to do, so in the end I kept the medal, but out of sight, so no one would know I had it. I wasn't fooling myself. I knew I hadn't earned it. Don was right. Looking back now, I think Shaaron Ackles tied me to that event that day as surely as if she had tethered me to the black rocks on the lava fields. Her heartfelt gesture proved I was part of the Ironman family and it sealed my fate. Before I left her office I knew I would be back again next year.

On my return to Australia I was again struck by the anticlimax of homecoming. I was living two separate lives—one here and one overseas—a world apart. I'm sure it didn't help that Cynthia and I had decided to go our own ways, although we hadn't ruled out the possibility of a reunion at some stage in the future. Long-distance relationships are difficult at the best of times, but I was in the middle of trying to achieve something that required about as much commitment as I could give.

In 1995 it had taken months for my body to recover from the punishing workout I'd given it in Hawaii. In 1996 I took four weeks off before getting straight back into training. I credit the quicker recovery to the more thorough preparation I had to begin with and to experience, which is a great teacher. I was now determined that 1997 would be my year. It would be third time lucky and I was going to give myself every chance of achieving what I had set out to do.

If anyone had asked me years ago whether I would go to

Hawaii a third time running to try to make the cut-off times, I would have said to them, 'You're dreaming!' It was the furthest thing from my mind. In retrospect it's probably the best decision I ever made. It gave me the confidence later on to stand before anyone and say, 'Don't give up. Sometimes you don't get it right the first time. But keep going, keep chasing your dreams because the journey is just as important as the destination.'

I didn't know for sure whether I would ever achieve what I wanted. I believed I could do it. I believed it would happen. I visualised myself at the finish line of that race with a medal around my neck, properly earned and proudly worn. But I also knew that life doesn't always pan out the way we want it to. But that doesn't mean we shouldn't try.

Before I flew home in 1996 I gave a talk to the Honolulu-based employees of Subaru, which was part of my sponsorship deal. Again I was struck by the impact my story had on everyone. Afterwards one of the local managers, Dennis O'Keefe, suggested I get in touch with a guy called Tony Garnett in Sydney. Tony, he said, might be able to help me. I didn't think much about it until early the next year, when I received two phone calls in quick succession over lunch. One was from Dennis in Hawaii, the other from Don in Canada. Both asked if I'd called Tony Garnett yet and when I said sheepishly, 'No, I haven't', they urged me to get on with it! I took it as a sign and called.

I went to see Tony at his Holden dealership and gave him the spiel: my life story, the rundown on my two previous attempts at making the cut-off times and my dream of being third time lucky in 1997. Tony sat in silence until I was finished, then said: 'I like you, Maclean, you're a bit of a mongrel. I want to give you a leg up.' Tony fascinated me. His contact book was like a *Who's Who* and he had a heart as big as Phar Lap's, and he was prepared to put himself out to help other people achieve their dreams. He had a plan: he would organise some of his friends to attend a presentation at Parramatta Leagues Club where I would be the guest speaker. We would see what developed from that.

No matter how much I try to rehearse lines or speeches, when it comes to delivering them to an audience they have a habit of developing a life of their own. Such was the case this day. I put together some slides and video clips from NBC's coverage of the 1995 Hawaii Ironman and with the help of these visuals spoke to a group of men and women I'd never met before but whose financial help I desperately needed.

My speech was well received, but I was surprised when people started approaching me afterwards with their business cards. I must have looked perplexed, because Tony intervened, smiling, saying he'd be my secretary. And that was it. On that day, on the back of a generous offer from a magnanimous man, I became a professional athlete. Sponsorship deals with companies like Holden, for which Tony was responsible, started coming my way and I had to pinch myself to make sure it was happening. I was almost thirty, and my boyhood dream of becoming a professional athlete had finally come true.

I started looking at the calendar and working out which events would be good to compete in. With some money in the bank I felt for the first time in years that I could be selective. In April 1997 I flew to Florida to compete in the St Anthony's Triathlon in St Petersburg. I was staying in a dingy hotel there when I met two English triathletes, Jason

Howard and Lee Hutchison, who recognised me from Hawaii and invited me to a barbecue that night. 'Do you want us to come and get you?' I said, 'That would be fantastic.' They turned up in a pickup, threw my wheelchair in the back—and that's how I met Karen and Robert Hoke, who were hosting the barbecue. By the end of the evening they had invited me to stay with them. They had a bunch of kids and a massive house and were involved in triathlons. It was perfect. I loved the company and the loving family atmosphere and they let me base myself there for the next six months.

The designer who'd built my racing wheelchair in 1995, Chris Peterson, worked not far from the Hokes. This time with no problems with finance, I went to see him about designing a new hand-cycle that would help me make up the minutes I needed to make the cut-off time for the cycle leg in Hawaii. We worked on a prototype together and then he built the bike from scratch. It was more aerodynamic and weighed only 9 kilograms.

While I was working on the bike with Chris another wheelchair athlete dropped in, Scott McNiece, who also lived in St Petersburg. Scott and I started training together. He was a double amputee and very strong on the hand-cycle, but I was faster in the wheelchair and a better swimmer. It was a bit of healthy competition for the two of us.

Convinced now that wheelchair athletes could successfully compete in the Hawaii Ironman, organisers announced that a new race category would operate from 1997—a wheelchair division. Three athletes would be given entry cards from the Buffalo Springs Half-Ironman in Lubbock, Texas, in June. It was game on! I wanted to be the first wheelchair athlete to make the cut-off times in Hawaii, but that now meant winning the category as well. I had never shied away from competition and thought it could work to my advantage—helping to push me harder—but it did up the ante. Suddenly more was riding on it, not least my pride.

I flew to Texas more determined than ever. Six wheelchair athletes had registered for the event. No longer was it simply a case of completing the course and qualifying. I had to finish in the top three. Apart from Scott, whom I'd competed against in a triathlon in St Petersburg and beaten, I had no idea about the pedigree of the other competitors. I started the race well and was first out of the water in the swim leg, but completely ran out of juice in the bike leg. Scott overtook me on the last big hill before the transition into the half marathon. I thought, 'I'll pick him up in the run', but physically I was spent. Thankfully, I made it to the finish line in second place and another American, Randy Cadell, came third. Scott was excited by his win and rightly so. He'd proved that he was a contender and I knew I'd have to do better in Hawaii if I were to beat him.

I boarded the flight back to Florida feeling disappointed, but relieved at the same time. I had qualified and at that stage that was all I had to do. I believe that it's important athletes move on quickly from their poorer performances and not get stuck on those less-than-perfect moments that can quickly lead to self-doubt. I was already gearing up mentally for my next race against Scott. I was confident I could improve— but I knew that both he and Randy had a lot more to prove than I did.

I can't say I was lonely, at least as far as female company was concerned. It was two years since Michelle and I had separated and she was also seeing someone else at the time, a fireman. But I couldn't help wondering about the possibility of reconciling. On many levels we were the perfect match. We had a shared history and a deep understanding of each other and I missed that. I missed her. I'm a sucker for happy endings, so I rang her and said, 'It's up to you whether you want to come over or not but you're probably wondering what I've been doing all these years and I'd like to show you.' I offered her a return ticket to Hawaii to watch me compete. I wanted her to witness the scale of the event and my involvement in it. I thought that then she might understand what it was I had been chasing since the accident. She agreed to come.

I like to assemble a team for these big events. One of the main reasons is the positive energy force it gives me. A friend once warned me, 'John, you are putting yourself under a lot of pressure doing that.' He was right, of course, but in a way I think having people around that I care about makes me want to achieve my goals even more. If I can see them in the crowd the last thing I want is to disappoint them.

As well as Michelle, I asked Dad to fly over. It was his seventieth birthday and I thought the trip would make a great present. It was my way of thanking him for all the time and effort and love he gave me over the years, but in particular after the accident. Dad was always 'Mr 100 Per Cent' and I learned a lot from him about putting maximum effort into the pursuits I cared about. He was delighted. The final member of the team was the ever-reliable Don. He flew in from Canada again to organise the race logistics and to run the sponsorship side of Team Maclean.

The day of the race drew nearer and I felt calm. 'My time has come,' I told myself over and over. I had paid my dues on this course and had learnt the lessons it had taught me in a tough love sort of way. I deserved this and nothing was going to stand in my way, certainly not two other wheelchair athletes.

Scott never trained with me after the half-Ironman in Texas. He didn't say why not but I think he thought he had the upper hand after beating me. A shift had occurred in our relationship, but looking back now I think that was a good thing. I don't think we should have trained and hung out together. We were in competition. Scott and Randy were both good guys. But I wasn't here in Hawaii to be their best friend. I was here to beat them and become the first wheelchair athlete in the history of the event to make the cut-off times and in the process win the category in its inaugural year.

I believe some people are meant to appear in your life at just the right time.

When I first competed in Hawaii the scene at the start of the race overwhelmed me. This year I soaked up the atmosphere but stayed focused. There were two volunteers to carry me into the water and then out of it and on to the transition area. By now all the volunteers were not only comfortable with wheelchair athletes, we were their favourite competitors. Lew Friedland told me recently, 'The best job in Hawaii with the race now as a volunteer is to get to work with the challenged athletes whereas before we couldn't get anyone to do it.' I take a great deal of pride in that. A large part of breaking down barriers involves educating people, and I loved being a part of that process.

I was nervous before the race, but as soon as I heard the cannon I was off. I had worked on my stroke in training and had swum a lot of kilometres over the preceding months that helped build up my endurance and ultimately my speed. I concentrated now on keeping up a strong, easy rhythm. I knew the course intimately and moved quickly through the water, conscious of not getting caught up with the other athletes. I was in the zone and before I knew it was at the finishing line after recording my best time in three years. I completed the leg in 60 minutes. The professionals do it in the high 40s, early 50s, so I was feeling confident. I was also in front of Scott and Randy and thought to myself, 'Okay, it's really game on now. Let's go!'

The cycle leg had twice before been the make-or-break part of the race for me. I hadn't made the 5.30 pm cut-off either time, defeated by my inexperience and the extreme conditions in 1995 and that ill-timed flat tyre in 1996. This year there was the added pressure from the presence of Scott and Randy. Scott, in particular, was strong in this leg, and I knew if I could hold onto the lead over the 180 kilometres there was a chance the Queen K might break his spirit, just as it had almost broken mine in 1995. I headed out quickly, knowing I didn't have a moment to spare. I had no idea how far behind the other two were and wouldn't know until either I turned around and came back up the Queen K or they overtook me. The latter thought was unacceptable and I started cycling harder.

I believe some people are meant to appear in your life at just the right time. Gordon Bell is one of those guys. A fellow member of the Nepean Triathlon Club, he was the athlete who hailed down the heckler giving me a hard time over wearing a wetsuit in 1995. I hadn't seen Gordon since then, until he miraculously turned up behind me on the Queen K this day. As he was overtaking me he shouted some words of encouragement that were like a shot of adrenalin pumped directly into my veins: 'You're flying, John. You're miles ahead of the other guy, you're going great, keep it up.' And with that he disappeared over the horizon. It was just what I needed to hear and I could feel my heart rate picking up as I sought to drive home my advantage.

I rounded the halfway point and started heading back up the Queen K, all the time thinking, 'Where are they? What position am I in?' I passed Scott heading for the halfway point some time later, and knew immediately I had a comfortable lead—but I couldn't afford to let my guard down. I was the last person in this race who needed to be told that things go wrong when you least expect them to.

As I approached the transition area for the start of the marathon, I could hardly stop myself from peering at the sun and gauging its position in the sky. I knew I had made better time this year, but I wouldn't—couldn't—allow myself the luxury of thinking I had it in the bag. When I finally cycled in, I relaxed enough to hear news that was music to my ears, 'John, you've made the cut-off time for the cycle leg.' Not only had I made it, I had 90 minutes to spare. Don was there to greet me with the biggest smile on his face. He helped me into my wheelchair. 'Giddy-up,' I thought. 'Let's get this job done.'

My new racing wheelchair was faster than my old one, and a completely different design. Instead of my legs being positioned in front of me, with my feet resting on a footplate, my legs were tucked up behind me. I'd been training in this position, which helped me generate greater power and thus more speed. People on the side of the road were clapping and cheering me on as I passed by, and a guy started yelling, 'You are the world champion!' I'm thinking, 'Take it easy, buddy!'

Throughout the race I'd been drinking lots of water and consuming carbohydrate gels—better known as goo—but now I ran out of supplies. I started consuming an energy drink available at the aid stations, which was a mistake, because the drink didn't agree with me. About a third of the way into this leg I started vomiting. The nausea swept over me like a tidal force. 'No,' I pleaded silently. 'This can't be happening.' I felt my energy flagging.

My pace slowed, but I kept moving, one turn of the wheel after another. I knew Scott and Randy could quickly make up ground on me and I had to maintain momentum. 'Just keep going,' I told myself. I had come too far to lose now. When the twinkling lights of Kona appeared on the horizon I knew I was home. Nothing short of a natural disaster would stop me now.

As I turned into Alii Drive the spectators went wild. I took off my gloves, pulled out my Australian flag and crossed the finish line in a time of 12 hours and 21 minutes. I had finally achieved what I set out to do, and had beaten a third of the field in the process. I didn't appreciate it fully at the time, but I had written myself into the record books of this event and something had finally clicked into place inside me.

For the first time since the accident I felt the equal of every athlete there.

CHAPTER TEN

SEE IT, BELIEVE IT, ACHIEVE IT

*'Not only was John an inspiration to other
challenged athletes but he was an incredible
inspiration to able-bodied people who fear not
being able to accomplish things ... He showed
the world things were possible that a lot of
people questioned'*
—LEW FRIEDLAND, FORMER PRESIDENT,
WORLD TRIATHLON CORPORATION

What I accomplished in Hawaii was special to me. But I didn't want just to go home with my medal and pick up the threads of my old life, nor did I want to compete in the Ironman again. It was time for a new challenge, time to up the ante. And soon I had a plan.

It was something I had been thinking about it since a guy called Ian Byrne introduced himself to me at the pool in Penrith, wanting to congratulate me on my sporting achievements. I had read about Ian in the local paper and knew he had just successfully swum the English Channel (at the age of forty-seven), so I returned the compliment of a job well done. 'Thanks,' he said. 'If I can do it, surely a young and sprightly thing like you can too.' (I was then thirty-two.) Ian later claimed he'd been baiting me that day, throwing down a challenge. I hadn't noticed because the idea was so intriguing it had completely dazzled me.

Swimming the English Channel is another of sport's Holy Grails. Only about 10 per cent of the endurance swimmers who tackle this infamous body of water between England and France make it across. I liked those odds, or I should say the challenge they presented. I liked the idea that I would be the first wheelchair athlete in history to have done it. Not only that, I would be the first athlete in the world—physically challenged or not—to have swum the English Channel *and* completed the Hawaii Ironman. 'How cool would that be?' I thought.

The prospect of being 'the first' at anything is a powerful lure to all athletes. How could it not be? Humanity is innately competitive. But while the possibility of having my name in the record books was attractive, it wasn't the only reason the idea flashed at me like a beacon on a dark night. Looking back, I think the validation I received from competing in the Hawaii Ironman made it almost impossible for me to stop at that. I was being noticed for all the right sporting reasons and I wanted that to continue.

Three years of competing in the Ironman had taught me a great deal about myself. I knew what made me happy and at that stage it wasn't a nine-to-five job, a nice house in a nice street and a good car. In many ways life would have been easier if I had been content with those. But I felt a burning need to push myself, to see how far I could go and what I could achieve despite being in a wheelchair.

Some people express themselves through music, some through art, some through their families. My way was sport. Maybe that fire in my belly ignited a long time ago when I was a little kid jumping up and down to get attention in Dalmar Children's Home. Maybe the accident added fuel to that fire because suddenly I had to fight to stay alive and to be noticed again for all the right reasons. Or maybe it was a combination of those things and the fact that I was born with sporting ability and the determination to succeed. I will never know, just as I will never know what would have happened if my life hadn't been turned on its head by the accident and I had continued playing rugby league. What I did know was that the fire was now burning so fiercely it was impossible to extinguish.

What had gone out, unfortunately, was the spark between Michelle and me. We couldn't make our relationship work. We tried. After the 1997 Hawaii Ironman we spent a few fabulous days together in a five-star resort at Kona and later, in Sydney, we went out a few times. But it was not to be. It was time to finally let go and I found it incredibly painful. It was one of the toughest lessons I've ever learnt. No matter how hard you work at a relationship, how much you might want it to succeed, if it's not meant to be, no amount of trying will change it. We both needed to move on.

Sport was a good distraction for a broken heart. I started planning my assault on the Channel. I contacted the now late, great Des Renford, the famous Australian endurance swimmer who made so many successful crossings—nineteen in total—that he became known as the 'Calais Commuter'. Des lived in Maroubra in Sydney's eastern suburbs and I went to see him with David Wells to hear first-hand just what I was letting myself in for and what I needed to do to take on 'the ditch'. I believe that going directly to the experts—the people with hands-on experience—helps save a lot of time and wasted effort. Des knew every pitfall and problem I would face and if there was a way of reducing the pain he would surely know it.

Since the late nineteenth century the Channel has been the greatest challenge for the world's long-distance swimmers. Des was very clear about its revered place in history: 'There is only one Wimbledon, there is only one Melbourne Cup, there is only one British Open, and in its purest form there is only one marathon swim in the world and that is to swim the English Channel.' But it's not easy. That's why swimmers wanted to do it. That's why I wanted to do it.

Des outlined the hazards—how quickly the water changes from being 'flat as a pancake' to a mountainous sea; how unpredictable the weather can be and what a big part the tides and currents play; how important it was to connect with an experienced boat captain who knew the waters—the Channel is the most congested shipping route in the world—and could pick the best possible time to undertake the crossing. It is about 32 kilometres in a straight line from the port of Dover in England, which is the main starting point for the crossing, to Calais in France, where most swimmers aim to finish. Rarely does anyone swim in a straight line, however. The tides and currents and treacherous winds have a habit of pushing swimmers off-course and adding many kilometres to the journey. If I were to make it, I would have to be prepared to swim between 40 and 90 kilometres.

Des addressed another issue that was on my mind—the devastatingly cold water I would be in for anything up to fifteen hours. According to the rules of the Channel Swimming

Association (CSA), the official body that supervises all crossing attempts, a swimmer can wear only a regular Speedo-type bathing suit, bathing cap and goggles. Grease or wool fat can be rubbed on the skin to help retain body heat, but a wetsuit—uh, uh—that was outside the guidelines and something the association was unlikely to agree to. Des was adamant on that point. This was going to be a problem. As well as warding off the cold, a wetsuit helped keep me buoyant. This was critical given the lack of movement in my legs and the fact they sank like anchors without a wetsuit. We did a bit of brainstorming and came up with the idea of strapping a flotation device between my legs to keep them up.

Des offered to put me in touch with a boat captain who he believed was among the best in the business. His name was Reg Brickell and his father, also Reg, had piloted the boat that shepherded Des on many of his crossings. Word-of-mouth recommendations like that are often the best kind of advice you can get, and I will always be grateful that Des was kind enough to share his contacts.

Shortly afterwards I contacted the CSA to formally apply for permission to attempt a crossing. I wanted it to be an official swim and was sure there would be some people on the committee who were concerned about safety and the ability of a wheelchair athlete to make the distance. I also needed approval to use the flotation device. My application had to go to a vote of a CSA subcommittee, a five-member panel, as it was classed as a special swim, and luckily for me three out of the five voted in my favour.

Training now started in earnest. I contacted the administrators of the Penrith Lakes seeking permission to use that body of water as my main training venue. Safety was their main concern. They said, 'If you've got someone to paddle next to you to keep an eye on you, that's fine.' For the next few months that person was Ian Morgan, who lived in the neighbouring suburb of St Clair. Ian had seen an article about me in the local paper and contacted me out of the blue offering himself as a training partner. As an avid sportsman himself, retired and thus available during the day, he was an ideal training partner for this new challenge. This always seemed to happen—just when I needed someone's help they would appear out of the blue. It was as if the script for my life had already been written.

Around this time another important person entered my orbit. David Knight would go on to become a critical figure in my Channel attempt, not to mention one of my best friends in the process. I had met David about twelve months earlier on the Sunshine Coast when I was competing in the Noosa Triathlon. Gatorade was a race sponsor and David was the company's new managing director in Australia. We met briefly at a lunch organised for athletes, sponsors and sports marketing executives and I liked him immediately. We didn't see each other again until late in 1997 when I ran into him on the steps of the Sydney Opera House with his wife Andrea, and their three young children. David was competing in the Noosa Triathlon that year—his first triathlon ever—and I agreed to do it too. We spent about a week together on the Sunshine Coast. David completed the course, which impressed me greatly given he hates training and is the first to admit it.

That night we went out to celebrate at the Rolling Rock Night Club. We got talking on the edge of the dance floor. 'I can't believe you've done Hawaii, that's amazing,' he said. 'What's next?' David is one of those warm and engaging characters with an open face and an inviting smile. 'I'm going to swim the English Channel,' I said without hesitation. 'What about you?' David ummed and ahhed for a few moments before he said, 'I'd like to do the Hawaii Ironman.' We still laugh about that night and how suddenly he went from competing in his first triathlon to committing to one of the world's toughest endurance races. 'That's the effect you have on people,' he told me recently. 'You raise the bar straight away.'

Sport wasn't our only bond. David and I had more in common than we first realised. His father had died when he was a young boy and I think being able to understand the loss of a parent and what that meant for a young kid growing up gave us a deeper connection, as did the fact we were both positive people who strongly believe life's too short to sit around complaining about bad luck. There are energy givers and energy takers in this world, and neither of us had time for the latter. It was obvious we were going to be good friends.

When I saw David the next day he slipped his business card into my hand and said, 'Come in and have a talk to us about what it is you want to do.' A week later I wheeled into Gatorade's headquarters in Sydney ready to give my pitch. But when I looked around at the executives in the meeting room, I decided to do what I did best—speak from the heart. I kept it short and simple. 'I'm here to get your support,' I said. 'For my next venture I plan to swim the English Channel and I'd like you guys to do a documentary or something else along those lines. I'm not asking for money for myself, but it would be nice to inspire kids in wheelchairs and show them that if I can do something like that they can do something too.'

David said, 'Okay, thanks very much,' and I left the room. I made my way to the elevator and just as the doors were closing

David popped his head in: 'You'll never know how much we got out of what you just said.' With that the doors closed, the elevator went to the ground floor and I left the building. It was the shortest pitch I'd ever made.

One of the best things about the media exposure I received doing the Hawaii Ironman was that I developed a profile, and more and more I was being asked to talk to kids in wheelchairs. My story and my sporting achievements made a real impact on them and for the first time in my life I was able to help people and give them hope that life goes on despite the challenges, that it is possible to achieve your dreams. Organisations were contacting me, as were families, schools and individuals. I thought the Channel swim was another great way of spreading the message that none of us should be defined by the wheelchair we use or the challenges we have—just by the size of the heart inside each and every one one of us.

I lucked out! Gatorade agreed to fund a documentary on my Channel swim and organise for it to be shown on national television. David must have sold the concept well because the investment the company made was around $100 000. I felt humbled by their show of faith and excited at the way momentum was starting to build. And there was more! David offered to be a support swimmer, which was incredibly generous given the training it would require him to do and the length of time it would take him away from his young family.

Under the CSA's rules athletes who attempt a crossing are permitted support swimmers. You must swim for the first two hours on your own but after that you can have a support swimmer with you every second hour. Support swimmers are incredibly important. They help maintain morale and monitor your mental and physical health. Ocean swimming—especially in notoriously rough stretches of sea like the Channel—can be daunting and I knew I needed all the help I could get. I was fortunate when another accomplished athlete and friend, Wally Brumniach, also volunteered to swim with me. Wally worked for a life coach called Maurie Rayner and was skilled in the power of positive thinking. Who better to encourage me along the way, especially when my energy levels flagged and my resolve weakened?

With my team assembled I felt confident I could overcome anything the Channel threw at me. I was about to enter a battle with Nature and I had no illusions as to which of us had the upper hand.

My training regimen was critical. I had to build my endurance and strength. I swam in the local pool and in the Penrith Lakes on weekdays and on Saturdays I would drive to Bondi, meet up with David Knight, and we'd plough through the water from south to north Bondi, up and back, up and back, rain, hail or shine. I gradually increased the distance, aware that I had to be as strong and fit as possible. It consumed my life and I was in the water six days out of seven.

I was confident I could cover the Channel distance. But even if I was lucky with the weather and the tides and the currents, I knew the painfully cold water would be a massive challenge. Many Channel swimmers had their dreams shattered because they couldn't handle the water temperature with just wool fat on their bodies for protection, and sooner or later became hypothermic. I went to see sports dietician Dr Helen O'Connor, who told me I had to beef up. 'If you don't put on weight you won't make it,' she said. 'You will get hypothermia. It doesn't matter how hard you try, John, you can't beat hypothermia.'

Dr O'Connor put me on a new diet—I had to put on fat. Long-distance swimmers carry a fair bit of excess weight and that's to protect them from the cold. I didn't really want to do this. I had always taken pride in being strong and lean. But I feared freezing and failing more than I valued my looks, so I dutifully starting eating more high-calorie food.

I downed a glass of orange juice and four slices of toast and honey before heading off to Penrith Lakes every morning. After swimming up to 10 kilometres I'd come home and have twelve Weetbix, a litre of full-cream milk, a can of fruit and another six pieces of toast with honey or jam. That was breakfast. I went to Penrith Plaza for morning tea—usually a large rum-and-raisin thickshake. For lunch I ate a pie or a couple of sausage rolls with hot chips, and in the afternoon I snacked on a chocolate éclair or custard tart washed down with coffee. I'd go home for a rest before heading out to the pool for another training session. For dinner I had a stir-fry of meat and vegetables with lots of rice, and I finished off the day with a family-size block of chocolate.

> One of the most valuable lessons I've learnt is not to worry about things I don't have control over.

Not surprisingly I started putting on weight despite all the swimming, piling on 20 kilograms. By the time I left for England I tipped the scales at 100 kilograms, the most I had ever weighed. I didn't like the way I looked. My rounded face and thicker frame were the worst part of the whole preparation. But I stopped looking in the mirror and told myself it was for a reason.

At that stage I didn't think I needed a swimming coach. I knew what I had to do and preferred the advice of people who had been there and done it, like Des Renford and Susie Maroney, who is still the only Australian to have successfully completed a double crossing in the one attempt. Susie was very encouraging and we did a couple of training sessions together and had long chats about what I could expect out in the Channel. A coach? No, I was doing okay—but as always fate had other ideas. I was swimming laps at the Penrith pool one afternoon when a guy came up to me and said, 'Hi, what are you training for?' I thought he was just being friendly. When I said, 'The English Channel', I could see him take a step back. His name was David Harvey and he was clearly intrigued by the ambitious goal I had set myself. David was an experienced swimming coach and joined our team not long after that— and I'm so glad he did. He worked on lengthening my stroke, which helped halve my stroke rate per minute and increased my speed at the same time. Being as efficient as possible in the water is important for endurance swimmers, and was more so for me because of a shoulder injury I was carrying. During the 1995 Hawaii Ironman I'd suffered a partial tear to the rotator cuff tendon in my left shoulder that had not fully healed. I was having regular physiotherapy treatment, but I was constantly aware of it.

As the winter approached I continued swimming in the Lakes. In the warmer months the water temperature was not a problem—I'd developed a terrific tan and thought 'This is groovy'. But as the season changed it was a different story. It got so cold that even Ian Morgan, who paddled beside me on his wave ski, started wearing a wetsuit and woolly hat—and he wasn't even in the water. At its coldest, the water dropped to

9 degrees Celsius, which was bone-chilling. I wouldn't have been able to handle it if I'd started training in that temperature, but swimming through the change of seasons meant that my body gradually acclimatised. I planned to swim the Channel in the northern hemisphere's summer when the water would be around 15 degrees Celsius. That was going to seem warm in comparison.

We started doing longer swims. The first was a four-hour stint at Penrith Lakes, which Wally and David Knight did with me, but we gradually lengthened the time until we were ready to tackle a twelve-hour swim up the Shoalhaven River on the New South Wales south coast. Dad came with us. It was dark for some of the time I was in the water and they had to keep a light fixed on me because otherwise they couldn't see past their noses. I wore a wetsuit on some swims and not others. On this outing wearing one proved to be a smart move. Late into the swim the boat's engine conked out, but I kept going. No one could see where I was and Dad was freaking out, concerned that I would get into trouble in the murky dark waters and never be seen again. Of course that didn't happen. They eventually got the engine started and caught up with me but I was oblivious to the drama.

Many people have asked if I felt scared in the unfamiliar salt waters I trained in while preparing for the Channel swim, especially of sharks. The simple answer is no, never. I could easily have died on the M4 twenty years ago. Every day since then has been a bonus. If I were killed tomorrow, I would like the world to know that I regarded myself as a lucky, lucky man for the extra time I was given on this earth. Some people call that fatalistic, and maybe it is. But fear is not something I feel. I think a lot of people do and their main fear is of dying. One of the most valuable lessons I've learnt is not to worry about things I don't have control over. When I was in hospital I yearned to be outside, looking at the sky and smelling the fresh air. I love the outdoors, but when it comes to Mother Nature I know who's the boss. I don't ever pretend I'm in control and that means I don't fear what's going to happen because I can't do anything about it. I felt that way about the Channel. It was a vast, unpredictable expanse of water whose mood was governed by tides and currents and weather patterns over which I had no control. I never felt frightened bobbing up and down in its depths, although I understand why some people get intimidated.

Some time earlier—well before my Channel preparations gained momentum and Gatorade agreed to fund the documentary—I signed a sponsorship deal with Nike. I had enjoyed a long relationship with the company, and its sports marketing people had always been supportive of my travails in Hawaii. It was a tricky situation because normally Nike does not co-brand, but Gatorade was funding the documentary and wanted branding of the boat that was piloting me on the swim. David Knight had to fly to Melbourne to meet Nike's sports marketing manager, George Lawler, to work something out. I needed every bit of support I could get and I was especially delighted when they reached a compromise in the interests of the documentary and sending a message to kids in wheelchairs.

Before I left for England, Nike called a media conference to formally launch my bid. On the day of the conference George presented me with a $20 000 cheque to put to a good cause. I know there are a lot of great charities out there but after thinking it over I decided to set up my own foundation. This was an important step and one I didn't take lightly. When we were growing up, Dad had always said, 'It's better to give than receive.' I agreed with that and for a while had been thinking about how I could give back to the community. It made sense to concentrate my efforts on what I knew—helping people who were physically challenged—and I loved working with kids. I wanted to raise money to help them and thought if I did it through my own foundation I could be more involved. That incredibly generous $20 000 from Nike kick-started the John Maclean Foundation and allowed us to help individuals who had a love of sport but didn't have the financial means to buy equipment like a racing wheelchair. After the presentation, the media took me out into the harbour because they wanted footage of me swimming with the Opera House in the background. I think if I were ever going to be taken by a shark that's probably when it was most likely to happen. They made me do it several times until they got their shots, and I laugh about it to this day. It was a glorious send-off and I enjoyed the attention and the focus it gave wheelchair athletes and what we can achieve if we set our minds to it.

Now the time came to leave for England. I had swum 1800 kilometres in training, and when I arrived in Dover for the final stage of my preparation I was pleased I had clocked up every single one of them. As I looked out towards the distant landmass I knew was France I took a deep breath. The enormity of what I had taken on suddenly hit me.

My support team started flying in from all over the world. David Knight was with me from the start, carrying me into the water for some last-minute training sessions so we developed a feel for the sea, which is a lot saltier than what we are used to in Australia. Wally Brumniach arrived with his wife Natalie;

David Harvey; my sister Marion; my brother Don with his two children Sean and Megan; my photographer friend Lisa Saad; and George Lawler from Nike. Cynthia and I had rekindled our relationship, and she flew in from Florida. Then there was the three-person film crew, shadowing my every move. Everyone was in place. It was now up to the Channel and Mother Nature when the crossing would get underway.

All the boat captains who guided Channel swimmers were fishermen. They knew the tides and currents and could read the weather patterns to pick the best time to go for it. I depended a lot on Reg Brickell and his seafaring expertise. He couldn't give me an exact date and time for the swim until a few days out, so I was sitting around waiting and hoping it would happen sooner rather than later. 'Bring the day on and let's do it,' I said to David Knight, who was coordinating the film crew and was just as impatient. On 15 August we got the call—we were up in two days' time. I was pleased it was finally locked in, but if people were expecting smiles and jokes from me they were sadly mistaken. David was right when he said, 'I knew you were thinking about the enormity of the challenge.' How could I not? I knew what lay ahead because I was looking straight at it.

At 6 am on 17 August 1998, I boarded *The Viking Princess* at the docks at Folkestone and said goodbye to Natalie, Lisa, Cynthia, Don, Sean and Megan. There wasn't room on the boat for everyone so they had to wait on shore. We headed out to Shakespeare Beach, where I was to officially start my attempt. David Harvey applied the wool fat en route, but apart from some general, good-natured banter, there wasn't much left to say. Under the CSA's rules I could not be carried into the sea. Once the starter's horn had sounded I had to make my own way from the high-water mark on the beach—and that meant turning around backwards and bum-shuffling down to the water across the pebbles and rocks. It amused me that they made no concession on this point, but in many ways I preferred it. The water was about 15 degrees Celsius, as predicted, much warmer than what I had been training in, but still cool enough to jump-start the adrenalin that was now coursing through my body. I gave a final thumb's-up and started swimming.

The first few hours were difficult. I lost some time at the start because a bit of wool fat got smeared on my goggles and I had trouble getting it off. I finally gave up and asked for a new pair. I was trying to find my rhythm but as always on a long-distance swim that was taking a while.

Every twenty minutes David Harvey would lower a Gatorade bottle attached to a nylon rope on the end of a broomstick into the water. I popped the top and consumed the contents as quickly as possible. Long-distance swimmers train themselves to go into a sort of meditative trance that not only helps pass the time but also 'takes them out of their bodies'. Some people talk about being able to look down at themselves and offer words of encouragement. I liked to imagine I was on a tropical island but it was hard to get this picture going, especially after the wind sprang up and the skies turned dark.

About six hours in, the water started getting rough. Reg, trying to position the boat to protect me from the tide and gusting wind, was growing increasingly concerned about the possibility that I'd drift into the side of *The Viking Princess* and hit the propeller at the back of the boat. He wanted to call it off. 'You've got to get him out,' he told David Harvey. I knew the weather had deteriorated, but I could still make out the French coastline on the horizon. 'I can still do this,' I told myself. I couldn't contemplate failure. Everyone had gone to so much trouble to get here, not to mention Gatorade's sizeable financial commitment. Who would want to see a documentary on a paraplegic not succeeding in swimming the Channel? What message would that send? All of these thoughts were swirling in my mind when David relayed the message. I replied, 'I want to go on.'

The CSA places an observer on each boat to ensure all swims go by the book. Norman Trusty had joined us on *The Viking Princess*, and he was clearly concerned. He thought I had lost valuable time at the start trying to clean my goggles and that I was taking food too regularly. But he liked my spirit and told the film crew, 'He's got all the guts I've ever seen for a swimmer out here. I hope he makes it.'

Against Wind and Tide was the title of the documentary and it couldn't have been more apt. The wind was indeed belting against the tide—and causing a frighteningly large swell. For three more hours I bobbed around like a bottle-top in a washing machine, trying to stay focused and positive but aware that time was slipping away. Channel swimmers must time their swims to coincide with the current that runs along the French coast, otherwise it's almost impossible to make it to shore. I needed to pick up the pace, but I was going nowhere.

Even Wally and David Knight, who had been upbeat and encouraging to this point, were becoming increasingly concerned. After finishing his hour-long turn in the water, David commented how frightening it was looking back into the boat, which at one stage tilted so far sideways he could see straight into the cockpit. At the nine-hour mark Reg, who had been closely monitoring the weather forecasts, came to the railings and told me I was going backwards, that I had not made any ground for the past three hours. 'You're not going to get anywhere, John,' he yelled down at me. 'No one can get across today. It's not you, it's the conditions.'

The fact that I had not made any headway for three hours broke my heart. There was no point continuing, so reluctantly I agreed to call it off. I swam to the rubber dinghy hanging off the stern of the boat and with what little strength I had left clambered in. From there David Knight hoisted me into the *The Viking Princess*, which was not easy given the now gale-force wind and churning sea. I was physically exhausted and emotionally devastated. David wrapped me in towels and rubbed my shoulders and legs to try and warm them up. I said nothing to anyone for a long time. I just sat there, shoulders hunched, trying not to think about anything, let alone the beating I had just taken from Mother Nature. The film crew, green with seasickness, were clinging to the fishing nets, trying to get some final bits of footage.

David strategically placed a towel with the Gatorade branding around me, then George stepped in with his Nike towel. I had to smile. Even with the attempt over, it was great to see a bit of healthy corporate competition. I admired them both for their dedication to their respective brands as the boat was flung about in the vicious sea. It took us hours to get back to Folkestone, and none of us said much because there was nothing much to say.

It was close to midnight by the time we reached shore. All the gear had to be unloaded and I huddled in the car with a tracksuit on trying to keep warm. All I wanted was a hot bath. When we finally made it back to the hotel at Dover, George tried to scrape the wool fat off me with a ruler. I was exhausted. I still remember the exquisite feeling of the warm water as I sank into the bath. I downed a cup of tea and went to bed.

The next morning I said to David Harvey, 'I want to give this another go.' He agreed, but it wasn't our decision. We didn't know if Reg could schedule us in again or whether he was fully booked for the rest of the swim season. We drove over to Folkestone to see him. 'I'd really like to have another crack at this,' I told him, half pleading. 'You've got all the heart I've ever seen,' he said. 'If we can slot you in we will but it won't be for a couple of weeks.' Obviously the rest of our team couldn't wait around for that long. Apart from David Harvey, they left, all pledging to return if they could reschedule their lives should we get another opportunity.

It's a mental game and you must believe in yourself otherwise when the going gets rough—when you're hurting and absolutely sick of it—you're not going to make it.

David Knight flew back to Australia. So did Marion and George. Wally and Natalie took off in a hire car to visit relatives in Croatia. Don and his children returned to Canada. Cynthia went back to Florida. Lisa left and so did the film crew. David Harvey and I began a nervous wait to see if I would get a second chance. For the first week I did nothing but eat and sleep, I was so tired. In the second week we found a physiotherapist who starting working on my shoulder. David studied the tides and we did some light training sessions. We decided I should shorten my stroke, which meant there would be less stress on my shoulder. I couldn't help thinking how fortunate I'd been coming across David. I hadn't been looking for a coach and he hadn't been looking for an athlete, but it turned out to be a perfect relationship.

At the end of the two weeks I got a call from Reg. 'You're going to get your second chance,' he said. I was booked in for 30 August, when the weather looked promising. 'We'll meet you at the dock at 4 am,' Reg said. I was ecstatic and started ringing around the team. Marion, Cynthia, George, Sean and Megan couldn't make it, but everyone else dropped everything and headed back to Dover, even the film crew, who had to jump on a long-haul flight from Australia.

I had never expected David Knight, who was on a skiing holidaying with his family at Thredbo in southern New South Wales, to return, but I rang him to tell him what was happening. 'What are you talking about?' he said. 'I'm on my way.' He packed up his family, drove the six hours back to Sydney and jumped on the first plane for London. It was going to be tight. The second time I spoke to him he had just arrived in Bangkok. I said, 'I've got to go at that scheduled time. I can't wait for you, mate.' David's plane was landing at Heathrow where he hoped he'd be able to hire a helicopter to drop him overboard into the Channel. As if that was going to happen! He would have to find some other way.

Meanwhile David Harvey and I had come up with a new game plan. I was only going to stop for food once an hour for the first three hours and then every thirty minutes after that, not every twenty. I wanted to put as much distance between me and the English side of the Channel as quickly as possible. We had a greater sense of what we were in for and I said to David, 'No matter what it throws at me, I'm getting to the other side.' The morning arrived and I knew I had to stay focused. Unlike the fanfare and cheery farewell of a couple of weeks earlier, our departure this time was more like a covert operation conducted in the pitch black. I had to enter the water bum-shuffling down from the high-water mark again, and I felt a slight sense of foreboding as I began to stroke through the water that looked like black oil in the dark.

I put my head down and went for it from the start. Marathon swimming is lonely. Even though you have support swimmers, they can't do it for you. It's a mental game and you must believe in yourself otherwise when the going gets rough—when you're hurting and absolutely sick of it—you're not going to make it. Both David and Wally were shouting out encouragement, 'You're making good time, you're doing great, keep going!' In the absence of David Knight, David Harvey stepped in as my second support swimmer. I had no idea where David Knight was and whether he'd even made it to England. But I appreciated him trying. I was searching for things to distract my mind, and when I saw my brother Don sitting in the cockpit of the boat, watching Formula One on television, eating a piece of cake and having a cup of tea, I thought, 'That would be right. Is he having one teaspoon of sugar or two?'

Unknown to me, David Knight was undertaking his own endurance event. He'd arrived at Heathrow after a delay in Bangkok, hired a car and driven in record time to Dover—and missed us by two hours. Having been told the helicopter plan was not going to happen (you're not allowed to drop people out of a helicopter into the middle of the Channel unless you're in the military), he ran up and down the docks desperately searching for someone with a boat who could take him out to try to find us. It was Bank Holiday and every available craft was out on the water. Eventually he found two young fishermen and told them his story. 'I've got a mate and he's in a wheelchair and he's swimming the Channel and I have to find him!' They looked at him like he came from Mars, but agreed to help when he pulled several hundred pounds from his wallet and said, 'You can buy a lot of fish with this.' They were still pretty dubious, and told him they only had two tanks of fuel. One was for the way out, and when it was empty they'd have to turn around because the second tank was for the return trip.

David was trying to stay in touch with *The Viking Princess* via two mobile phones—one was his and the other he'd borrowed from the guy who ran the bed and breakfast where the film crew was staying—and the boat's radio, but it was erratic and unreliable. To make matters worse his mobile ran out of battery and the other ran out of coverage. It was now like trying to find a needle in a haystack. Even more frustrating, the fishermen had just bought a Global Positioning Satellite system but didn't know how to work it. David was tearing his hair out. 'It was a fiasco,' he told me later.

The first fuel tank was running low and the fishermen were becoming anxious. 'It's time to turn back,' they said. David had convinced them to stay just a little bit longer when the radio suddenly crackled to life. From *The Viking Princess* Reg was saying, 'We're next to the ferry!' Normally that would mean nothing because there might be ten ferries on the Channel at any one time. But at this moment there was only one—right in front of the fishing boat. And there next to it was *The Viking Princess*. The fishing boat came alongside and David scrambled on board. He was wearing his wetsuit under his clothes and stripped off before perching on the side railing. I must have sensed his presence because for the first time I looked up and there was David saying, 'Hello mate.'

It was one of the most amazing moments of my life. I had no idea how he'd managed to find us in the middle of the Channel, but I was so glad he did. 'I've got the best friends in the world,' I thought, and with that put my head down and started swimming again. My arms felt lighter. I'd been swimming for six hours but now I'd just received a bolt of energy that I knew had come straight from my heart. David's appearance had renewed my faith that yes, I *would* make the crossing this day. How could I not after all that he—and the others—had done for me?

I'd like to say it was smooth going from there, but swimming the Channel doesn't quite work like that. It was a good day for it but I knew I had to keep up the pace. If I didn't properly time my attack on the French coast I could get caught in the tide and the current and I wouldn't make it to shore.

Reg stuck his head over the side and said, 'You need to pick up the pace. You've still got to get across the current and if you don't you won't make it.' By now I had been in the water more than twelve hours, my shoulder was aching and I was exhausted. That's the cruel nature of this swim. Just when you're at your most vulnerable you must find something extra within to finish it. The last kilometre was make or break. 'Pick it up, Johnno!' they started yelling from the boat. 'Pick it up!' I started swimming as hard as I could, drawing on every last ounce of strength I possessed. 'I can do this,' I kept telling myself.

It's amazing how long swimming one kilometre can take when you are fighting a powerful current. I knew if I didn't push myself to the limit I'd be washed away and would have to wait for the tide to change before trying again hours later. I think it was that thought that forced me to keep going. I couldn't fail. I just couldn't. Too much was at stake for too many people.

When I finally made it across the current and into the shelter of the bay, the environment changed completely. The water was warmer, the air was warmer, the sun had broken through the clouds and seemed to be shining as if personally welcoming me to France. David Knight was swimming alongside me. He told me later he was thinking, 'We're here, it's finally done, we've made it.' Then I stopped. He looked at me in horror: 'What's wrong?' 'I just want to savour the moment,' I replied.

I gave him a hug and said, 'Thanks for your support.' I don't know if that was allowed under the rules, but I have the certificate now that says I successfully swam the English Channel and they can't take it away from me. I swam into shore and as I was making my way across the pebbles and sand, bum-shuffling up to the high-water mark, I picked up some pebbles and stuck them down the front of my Speedos. Someone else I knew who had swum the English Channel recommended doing that so I had a keepsake of the experience. I collected four pebbles—which I still have—and while I didn't know it at the time they served another purpose. When I finally made it to the high-water mark, signalling the end of the swim, I fell backwards on the beach with the biggest smile on my face. Courtesy of those pebbles, the photos made me look very well endowed.

Captain Mathew Webb was the first person to swim the Channel. He breast-stroked across on 25 August 1875 in 21 hours and 45 minutes and later declared, 'Nothing great is easy.' It had taken me 12 hours and 55 minutes to become the first wheelchair athlete in history to make the crossing, and I did it one stroke at a time. I agree with Captain Webb's sentiment.

CHAPTER ELEVEN

FINDING HOPE

'Life is pretty short and I don't have time—and neither does John—for negative people. There are energy givers and energy takers and John is a big energy giver. He's very positive, everything is possible'

—DAVID KNIGHT, BEST MATE

N o one watching my struggles to swim a mere 25 metres in the hydrotherapy pool at Royal North Shore Hospital could have imagined that I would one day swim the English Channel—yet ten years later, on 31 August 1998, I woke up having achieved exactly that. I was utterly exhausted and my shoulders ached so much I could barely move, but I didn't care one iota about the pain. I felt so exhilarated I knew it would take weeks to come down to earth.

When we got back to Dover aboard *The Viking Princess* we celebrated with champagne—in plastic cups. In truth I was more interested in a warm bath and a soft bed, but it was great to share the moment with my friends and family. We packed up our gear the next day and said thank you to Reg Brickell.

Most of the team left; they had put their lives on hold and it was time to get back to the real world. David Knight, David Harvey, Don and I went to London, where a friend of David Knight's, who worked for Pepsi, took us out for dinner. We went to a swanky restaurant where the food was exquisite and every place setting had five glasses. In the space of a few days I had gone from Gatorade and goo to sampling some of the finest wines in the world and lamb that tasted nothing like the roast lamb I had for dinner when I was a kid.

I will never forget where I came from. I loved my childhood in western Sydney and it remains an intrinsic part of who I am today. But I couldn't help thinking this night about just how far I had come in life. I'd never envisaged fine dining in London or some of the other experiences I'd been lucky enough to enjoy. Putting up my hand for the Hawaii Ironman and swimming the Channel had expanded my horizons beyond my wildest imagination.

When I mentor people I press home this point. 'Don't be frightened to set goals, however audacious they might seem,' I say. Sometimes they question me: 'What if I don't achieve my goals? What then?' I tell them I am living proof that things don't always work out how you planned, but life goes on regardless. If you don't put yourself out there, however, nothing will ever happen.

After the Channel swim I felt really confident. I was only thirty-two, and I knew there was a lot more I could achieve in sport. I came home believing I had beaten my demons and enjoying the notoriety my overseas exploits attracted. I had no idea, however, of the turmoil that lay ahead or the ghosts in my past I was yet to confront. I didn't know it at the time but I had not grieved those cataclysmic events that changed the landscape of my life—my birth mother's psychiatric illness and the fact I'd never connected with her emotionally; the accident and what it had robbed me of; and the breakdown of my marriage. I thought I had dealt with these issues but I hadn't. If I had known what lay ahead of me, maybe my choices at that stage would have been different. Like many other men I might have turned and bolted, or reinforced the wall I'd rebuilt around myself in the months after the accident. But I was oblivious to the collision course I was on and kept on doing what I always had—thinking about my next sporting challenge.

A couple of months after I got back the documentary chronicling my Channel crossing, *Against Wind and Tide*, was launched in Sydney at a red-carpet affair in the city. It was well received and later aired on national television. I had been nominated for the NSW Athlete of the Year in 1997 and then, to my delight, again in 1998. I didn't win on either occasion, but the recognition by my peers was reward enough.

Cynthia had come to Sydney and moved in with me, and we were giving our relationship the chance to move to the next level. It must have been difficult for her relocating in a new city in a different part of the world. When we lived together in Florida I was training six days a week and had a goal I was working towards. I think she found moving to Sydney challenging, like starting afresh, but I wasn't in the right space to help her adjust. It wasn't long before we were rethinking whether cohabitation was such a good idea. Three months later Cynthia was on the plane back to Florida and I was again using sport to fill an emotional vacuum. I was also working hard to lose the weight I'd gained for the Channel swim—and once again I had a plan.

Some athletes define themselves by dominating one sport, as Lance Armstrong did with cycling; others by one event, as Des Renford did with the Channel swim. Neither of these approaches appealed to me. I wanted to try my hand at different sports, just like when I was a kid and I wanted to taste all the flavours in the ice-cream shop. A good friend once said to me, 'John, whether you know it or not, you're a conqueror.' He meant I liked to set myself a challenge, achieve it, and then move on to the next. He was right, of course. And in the end the diversity of sports I mastered helped distinguish my sporting career. But it would be wrong to assume that was my plan from the beginning. It wasn't. I was following my heart, not my head.

Around this time, Sydney was gearing up to host the greatest show on earth, the 2000 Olympic Games, and straight after that the Paralympic Games. I didn't have to look far afield for my next goal. I wanted to represent my country in wheelchair racing and take my place at the starting line in the Olympic Stadium at Homebush with a home crowd cheering me on in the stands. I wanted to hear my name called over the loudspeaker and feel those butterflies fluttering in the pit of my stomach as I waited for the starter's gun. I wanted to be part of Australian history.

After the 1995 Hawaii Ironman I'd flirted with the notion of trying to make the basketball team for the 1996 Paralympics. In fact, I was chosen in the train-on squad for Atlanta, but withdrew when it became clear to me that I had 'unfinished business' in Hawaii and I simply had to try once again to make those cut-off times. But the idea of representing my country had never gone away; I was just waiting for the right time and the right opportunity to present themselves.

A foray into wheelchair racing seemed a logical move. I had spent a lot of time in my wheelchair competing in triathlons and the Ironman, and I thought I could adapt pretty quickly. I met a coach called Jenni Banks who agreed to train me, although she pointed out that I was facing an uphill battle. I was a novice in a sport with many experienced competitors and, while I had competed in three marathons as part of the Ironman, actual wheelchair racing was completely different. Jenni organised for me to compete in my first 10-kilometre race in Sydney on Australia Day 1999, and we agreed we'd see how I went before making any further plans. The race was to be staged in The Rocks, at the foot of the Sydney Harbour Bridge and the western shore of Sydney Cove. It is the oldest part of Sydney—and truly breathtaking. The race was called the Oz Day 10K, and boasted a stellar international field of fifty competitors. Jenni said if I could go around in about twenty-seven minutes that would be a pretty respectable time.

Because of the profile I had developed after the Hawaii Ironman and the Channel swim the press swooped, and an article appeared on my taking up wheelchair racing. I understood the newsworthiness of my move, and the fact that it generated some hype around the event, but I underestimated the noses that would be put out of joint by that article. Hierarchies develop within every sport and while I had been accepted into the triathlon community, some people in wheelchair racing weren't quite so welcoming.

I built a small but incredibly focused and positive team of people around me when I took on Hawaii and the Channel and I can't overstate how that contributed to my success in those events. People like Johnno and David Knight trained with me and encouraged me every step of the way. When I felt like giving up, their belief in my ability helped get me through. But in wheelchair racing I was largely on my own—and I have to admit I felt vulnerable for the first time in years. Rivalries develop in any sport, especially at the top level. All elite athletes want to win. But I wasn't prepared for the intensity of it in wheelchair racing. I was the new kid on the block and not everyone was happy that I was encroaching on their turf.

Nonetheless, the Oz Day 10K was an exciting race—and I was pumped from the start. I wanted to do well and to prove to myself, and everyone else, that I could master the sport and had the speed required to be competitive with the best. Ten kilometres sounds like a long distance but in a wheelchair it can be covered quickly. I put my head down and went for it, coming tenth and recording a time of twenty-six minutes, a minute better than Jenni's most optimistic prediction.

It was now game on! But to make the Paralympic team I had to qualify. Given I had no runs—or times—on the board, I was starting from scratch. Jenni and I thought it best if I tried out for a few different events—the 1500 metres, 5000 metres, 10 000 metres and marathon—in the hope that I'd make it through to at least one of them. I started training with 26-year-old Australian wheelchair racer Paul Nunnari in early 1999. Paul became a paraplegic after a car accident when he was only eleven, and was a lovely guy. We struck up a friendship straight away. Jenni was coaching us both and I thoroughly enjoyed the time we spent together on the track, on the road and in the gym.

The plan was to compete in as many races as I could, to try to equal or better at least one of the qualifying times. In effect, I was trying to ratchet up a lifetime of experience in the sport in less than eighteen months. I would be competing against racers who had been specialising in it for decades. They knew their equipment inside out and they knew about tactics, which play a big part in wheelchair racing. They knew when to make their move on the track and when to hold their ground. They also knew each other's strengths and weaknesses, which was another advantage because it gave them an insight into how a race might unfold on the day and when they should be countering an attack from another competitor. I was an endurance athlete, with stamina and determination. I was a quick learner and a natural competitor. But I knew I had a lot to learn.

Things don't always work out how you planned, but life goes on regardless. If you don't put yourself out there, however, nothing will ever happen.

As I had done previously, I turned to the experts to get as much information as I could about the sport. I made the train-on squad for the Paralympic athletics team in 1999 under national coach Andrew Dawes. That didn't mean I was on the team for Sydney, just that I was identified as a promising athlete and supported financially to travel overseas and take part in certain international meets. There were three wheelchair racers in the squad: 18-year-old Kurt Fernley (who went on to become a great racer, winning a number of medals in Sydney, in Atlanta in 2004 and in Beijing in 2008), my training partner Paul Nunnari, and me. We could only qualify at special international meets so my training regime had to be designed around them.

When I was overseas I sought advice from the best in the sport, including Heinz Frei, from Switzerland, who would be forty-one when he competed in Sydney—his sixth Paralympics—and had won a swag of gold medals already, earning himself the nickname 'Mr Marathon'; Saul Mendoza from Mexico, another legend and former gold, silver and bronze medallist; and Jeff Adams from Canada, a six-time world champion. They were prepared to share information with me because they were generous and comfortable in their own abilities—and aware of my inexperience. I wasn't expected to be competitive; I wasn't a threat. I was the Ironman and the guy who had swum the Channel; no one expected me to make the transition in time to make a big impact. I'm a great believer that if you ask the right questions of the right people, you'll get the right answers, so I bombarded them with everything I didn't know: 'What do you think about the size of a push rim? What's the best glove to use? What's your training regime?'

I was improving; my times bore witness to that. I was hopeful I would achieve my goal—to make the Paralympic team. I'd like to make a point here because it is an important one. My goal was not to win a gold medal in Sydney, or silver or bronze. I would have liked to, sure. But the goal I set myself was to represent my country and participate in the event. I believe, in hindsight, that I made a mistake in limiting myself to that. I'm not saying that if I had set my sights higher I would have achieved better results. But it taught me a valuable lesson. People, including athletes, rarely punch above their weight. By that I mean, if you don't believe you are good enough to win, or at least are in with a chance, then you are never going to get there. If you don't see it and believe it you won't achieve it. I made many mistakes in the lead-up to Sydney but that was probably the biggest. I aimed to be at the Paralympics— so I had already won my gold medal when I was eventually selected in the team.

When I tell people this story they often flinch and hesitate before asking me, 'What's wrong with setting a goal like making the team!' 'Nothing,' I reply. 'But I never really wanted to settle for just that.' Looking back now I realise I hoped for more, that the roar of the home crowd would inspire the performance of a lifetime and that I would win gold or at least be among the medallists. That can happen, but not often. Once I started recording good times at international meets and beating some of the guys I would be competing against in Sydney, I should have revisited my goal. I should have started visualising myself on the dais, not just getting to the starting line.

I spent a good deal of time overseas in the lead-up to 2000. Paul and I spent a month in Switzerland at the Swiss Paralympic Centre where Heinz Frei was based, and we did the Boston Marathon together in April 2000, where I came fourth, far exceeding my expectations and giving me real hope I was developing into not only a good racer but a worthy competitor. We competed in other events in the United States and in Canada, and when we weren't overseas we were training together at Penrith. Eventually I qualified for the 1500 metres, 5000 metres, 10 000 metres, marathon and the 4 × 400-metre relay team. I was on my way to the Paralympic Games.

Around this time I received a phone call from Chris Nunn, the head coach of the Paralympic athletics team. He told me there was going to be a demonstration 1500-metre wheelchair race at the actual Olympic Games. Because Australia was hosting the Games a green card would be allocated for one

Australian male to participate. No qualification was needed. The female spot had already been allocated. I felt my heart beat faster. Was it possible? Could I be the one? It seemed like a dream come true and I told Chris in no uncertain terms how interested I was in being that person. Chris said Kurt and Paul were also keen, and by the end of our conversation seemed to have changed his mind about allocating the card out of hand. In retrospect, it wasn't that surprising. Imagine having to choose? Instead, he said, we'd have to qualify like all the other competitors at an international meet closer to the Games.

The possibility took my breath away. I desperately wanted to be in that race so I ramped up my training and started focusing on qualifying. The meet to determine who would make it into the Olympic race would be held at Delémont in Switzerland: four heats and then two semi-finals. Eight competitors would go through to the final, and that was the race that would be staged in Sydney.

The three of us from Australia would have to produce the performances of our lives to make it through. The best wheelchair racers in the world were all in Delémont, all vying for the same thing. I drew Heinz Frei in my heat. He was the most accomplished racer in the world, but I told myself, 'He's only a man.' My tactics were clear—Heinz was a slow starter so I'd try to get to the front and stay there as long as possible. When he caught me I'd attempt to use his draft to take me to the line. Drafting is an important tactic in wheelchair racing. If you can tuck in behind another competitor you can let them do all the work and be carried along in the slipstream. All racers do it and the ones who do it best tend to get better results. My plan worked. I took the lead and, as predicted, Heinz caught me with about a lap to go. I nipped in behind him and tried to power on to the finish line. I came second. More importantly, I was through to the semi-final.

Kurt also progressed through his heat, but Paul didn't. I really felt for Paul. He was a great guy and a talented racer but some days it works for you and some days it doesn't. Competition racing is cruel like that. I tried to put his loss out of my mind and stay focused. The top three in each semi-final would make it through to the final, plus the two competitors with the best times after that. I didn't want to go right down to the wire so I aimed to finish in the top three. My race plan was the same as in the heat. Get to the front—and stay there. Every racer has their strengths. I had trained for so many years as an endurance athlete that mine was strength and stamina, not necessarily speed, so it made sense to be a frontrunner and make the others try to catch me. As we lined up for the start, I could feel the nervous energy flow through my body. 'This is it,' I told myself. 'It comes down to this.' The starter's gun went off and I surged to the front. One lap. Two laps. Three laps. Could I hold on? With 200 metres to go I was cut off by a racer who overtook me. I managed to swerve in time to avoid running into him and made it to the line in third place. I couldn't believe it. I had qualified for the Olympics!

I barely had time to enjoy the moment before I was told there was a protest. My heart sank when I heard I was at the centre of it. Apparently when I swerved to avoid the racer in front of me I had caused another competitor to crash behind me. I waited anxiously for the result, thinking, 'I can't believe this is happening.' It was like being given a gift I'd always wanted only to have it snatched out of my hands before I could open it. The verdict was both good news and bad. I wasn't disqualified, the racer who cut me off was, but the race would be re-run. One minute up, the next down. Racing is like that.

When we wheeled to the starting line again I felt composed. My tactics hadn't changed. The starter's gun went off and I bore down on the push-rims of the wheels with every ounce of strength I had. I wanted to get to the lead and let the others catch me. Again I was in front for the first three laps, throwing down the challenge to the others waiting to make their moves. When they did I had to be ready to surge for the line with everything I had left. With about 200 metres to go the pack edged closer. One competitor overtook me, then another. I could sense others closing the gap fast. 'Hold on, John,' I told myself. 'Hold on.' A third racer had drawn level with me. We crossed the finish line neck and neck in a photo finish for third. I think I held my breath for as long as it took them to post the result. I had come third by the smallest of margins. I had earned myself a berth at the Olympics.

It should have been one of the happiest moments of my life. And it was for a few, brief minutes. I was the only Australian to have qualified. I completely appreciated Kurt's disappointment (he didn't make it through his semi-final) and Paul's disappointment, and they were as gracious as they could possibly be under the circumstances. When I was in the team room afterwards, however, some of the others weren't so generous. One member of the squad approached me directly. I knew this person wasn't my biggest fan but I wasn't expecting what followed: 'It's okay for you—you had an accident and received money for it. You've only been in the sport a short amount of time and you're going to the Olympics. You've been in the papers and you haven't done anything.' I was completely taken aback. I tried to see it for what it was—jealousy and insecurity—but personal attacks, especially those fired as a bullet to the heart, are not easily deflected, especially when they are shot at close range.

I left the venue and went back to my accommodation. There were no celebrations or claps on the back for a job well done. There was no sharing the journey or enjoying the moment. I went to bed that night crying into my pillow. All I could think of was Avril. I wanted my birth mother, just like a little kid does when they've been hurt. I wanted someone who loved me more than anything to hold me and whisper, 'Everything will be all right.' Maybe the fact that I had never had that deep emotional connection made me crave it more than anything else at that point. Maybe I was experiencing grief for the first time—grief that I had no one to comfort me, grief that I had been hit by the truck, grief that life wasn't working out like I thought it should. I had learnt early on that running faster and jumping higher than anyone else brought me personal validation, but today that hadn't happened. 'This isn't how this should be,' I thought despondently. 'This is not what I pictured. It should be a highlight of my life and it's not.' I rang Michelle because I needed to hear her voice. She was the woman I had felt closest to in my life, and I needed desperately to be comforted. All I wanted was to come home and rid myself of the emotional pain that was enveloping me.

It is not my intention to dig up old grievances or to make excuses for what was to follow. I mention this encounter purely because it was seminal for me on a number of different levels, including the lessons I learnt from it. I had already felt on the outer with some of the squad before the meet. Now I felt genuinely isolated. The verbal attack triggered an emotional response that was both a surprise and a revelation. No one goes from not having thought about their birth mother for years to desperately wishing she were still alive unless there are some skeletons rattling around. I returned home to Australia as flat as a board and, perhaps more importantly, emotionally fragile.

My coach Jenni Banks was fabulous. Unfortunately she lived and worked in Canberra so she sent me my training regime by fax every week. The rest of the athletic squad trained with national coach Andrew Dawes, who was based in Sydney. Andrew was equally impressive and in hindsight I probably should have swapped coaches so there was someone around to advise on technique and provide encouragement during my training sessions. It also helped training with a squad. When Paul joined Andrew I was on my own except for one session a week when we all trained together. Did my wariness about contact with some of the squad members influence my decision? Probably. And that was a mistake. I should never have let conflict get in the way of my training. I think my times would have improved under Andrew's tutelage, but I didn't make the move, so I'll never know for sure.

The important thing I learnt from this was that conflict is part of life, regardless of whether it's on a sporting team or in an office. Inevitably there will be people who don't like you and that's okay. Could I have handled it better? Short of bringing the issue to a head and attempting a reconciliation, I don't think so, but I probably should have joined the squad. Then again, perhaps not—I lacked the emotional resilience at that stage of my life to cope with the personal issues involved. My self-worth was too tied up in how much I achieved in sport, and I was headed for a big fall, although I didn't know it at the time. I can't help but think all this was meant to happen to prompt a change in my life. But, as always, it was not going to happen subtly. I was a full-on sort of person who achieved spectacularly and failed spectacularly, and when the wake-up call came it was earth-shattering.

The lead-up to the Games was unbelievable. I was training hard, but it was impossible not to get caught up in the excitement pulsing through Sydney. I was given the honour of carrying the torch down my street in Penrith and I couldn't quite believe the magnetic quality of that cylinder and flame until I saw the way people flocked to it like bees to a honeypot. It was an amazing event to be part of and one of my favourite memories of the Olympic experience. I felt like I had come full circle in my life—from that eager 12-year-old who had won the national race-walking title twenty years earlier to the Olympic athlete set to compete on the world stage. I was also delighted to be able to share it with Kane Towns, the son of Ched Towns, my blind friend who'd been one of the groomsmen at my wedding and who'd died of a heart attack a few years earlier while climbing in the Himalayas. Kane grew up to be a fine young man and I know his father would have been terribly proud.

The wheelchair demonstration event was scheduled for 28 September 2000, thirteen days after the Games officially opened. I was stunned when I was asked to lead out the men's team at the opening ceremony with Kurt Fernley, whose time at Delémont had made him a late inclusion after one of the other competitors dropped out. Wheeling into the Olympic Stadium behind Australia's flagbearer, basketballer Andrew Gaze, and hearing the roar of the crowd was incredible. I had to pinch myself to believe I was part of it all. 'Remember this,' I told myself, 'because you'll never be back here.'

... conflict is part of life ... Inevitably there will be people who don't like you and that's okay.

I didn't stay at the Olympic Village the whole time, checking in only the day before our race. After the opening ceremony I returned to Penrith and continued training until the morning of the event, which was scheduled for 7 pm. I went into the Village, and at lunch in the food hall I ran into Herb Elliott, Australia's legendary 1500-metre runner. I asked his advice and he said, 'Get in front and stay there, it's always worked for me.' I took it as an omen because they were my tactics to a T. That's exactly what I planned to do.

As the event drew nearer I went to the warm-up track. I hadn't beaten most of the other competitors in the race, so I knew it would take an extraordinary performance to win a medal. But I was hoping the crowd could lift me. I have never entered a race I didn't think I could win, which speaks volumes about my competitive nature.

Wheeling into the Olympic Stadium was an amazing experience. It was a beautiful night—clear and mild—and the stands were packed with 115 000 people. When my name was called over the loudspeaker system, and especially when they announced my country of origin—Australia—the roar was so loud I was sure it must have been heard all the way to Penrith. Kurt's introduction attracted the same raucous reception. I sensed that if I were well placed at the finish the crowd might just get me over the line. I tried to enjoy the moment and take long deep breaths to steady my nerves and pounding heart. I focused on the starter's gun and the power I needed to generate immediately to get to the front of the pack. I had drawn lane 1, which meant I had to go out quickly or I ran the risk of being boxed in. As we waited for the gun I couldn't help but notice how quiet it was in the stadium. You could have heard a pin drop.

Everyone was waiting ... waiting ... waiting ... and then the gun went off and we were away. The crowd was going wild as I hit the push-rims as hard as I could. It was a 100-metre sprint to the first bend and an explosive start was critical. I had to be in a good position as we turned into the back straight because I didn't have the kick some of the other competitors had to overtake in the run to the finish line. As we flew down the track I tried to hold the lead but when we entered the bend I was jostling for outright second place with Canadian Jeff Adams. American Scott Hollenbeck was in the lead. I was hugging the inside lane, conscious of not falling back in the field. 'Hold your ground, hold your speed,' I kept telling myself as I concentrated on the position of my wheels and on my breathing. I held on as we rounded the bend into the back straight, and was clear in second place with Hollenbeck setting a cracking pace out in front. We completed the first lap in a fast 54.78 seconds. I was feeling comfortable, confident I was racing well within myself and had enough in reserve to be in the mix at the finish. I was keen to stay as close to Hollenbeck as I could as we powered around the track. Heinz Frei was leaving nothing to chance. Instead of his customary late finish he was pushing hard now. As we moved into the third lap Frei surged to the front. There was nothing in it. Jeff Adams had come up through the field and I had slipped back into fourth, but it was still anyone's race. No one was out of it. Kurt came up on my inside as we got the bell for the final lap. I was concentrating on making every stroke of the push-rim as clean and powerful as possible. South Africa's Ernst Van Dyck was coming up on my outside and with 300 metres to go we came perilously close to each other. As my arm came down it collided with Van Dyck's coming up, and I felt the wheelchair tip. As my body hit the track the crowd gave a collective groan of disappointment. I was out of the race.

I couldn't believe it. I sat on the track wishing the ground would open up and swallow me whole. I could feel thousands of eyes on me as an official raced across to check I was okay. Apart from a badly grazed left shoulder, which had connected at speed with the track, I was fine, at least physically. My pride, however, was another matter. No one could have scripted a more ignominious ending to a long-held sporting dream. 'Why me?' I thought. 'Why now? Why here?'

I couldn't shake the strangest sense of *déjà vu* that had suddenly overcome me. Sitting on the track, trying to keep my emotions in check, I felt I had been here before. It was as if I were looking down at an event that had already taken place and revisiting it at another moment in time. I hadn't hit my head, so I wasn't hallucinating, and I don't believe in religious epiphanies, so it wasn't that, but the feeling was too strong to ignore. It got me thinking, 'Is there a path or highway that we were all destined to go down and this just happened to be mine? Was I meant to crash at the Olympic Games?' If I was, I hoped there was a bloody good reason for it, because right now I was struggling to think what it might be.

I asked the official to help me back into my chair so I could finish the race, but that wasn't going to happen. I had to get off the track. Not only had I crashed in front of 115 000 people, most of them Australians who'd been cheering me on, hoping I'd win a medal, but a DNF would be recorded against my name.

Mexico's Saul Mendoza and Frenchman Claude Issorat came first and second respectively. They were both behind me when I crashed, which gives some indication of how you can never confidently predict the outcome. They'd allowed the rest of the field to do the work out front and had enough left to overtake the leaders at the end. Heinz Frei, who'd taken the lead just before I fell, came third.

I did what I had to do. During an interview after the race I hid my feelings. When asked how I was feeling I said, 'It's not the result I was looking for, but these things are part of wheelchair racing. Now I am looking forward to the Paralympic Games and doing the best I can.'

I went back to the Village and collected my gear. My mobile phone was filled with messages from friends and family. I spoke to Jenni, who reassured me it was a great achievement to even make the Olympics, especially as I had only taken up the sport so recently. I appreciated the sentiment, and knew it was heartfelt, but I had always hoped I would win. Crashing was never part of the plan, certainly not in front of my home crowd or an estimated television audience of 3.7 billion people worldwide. I felt overawed by the experience. But there was something else I couldn't quite put my finger on. I had invested so much of myself into my sporting pursuits that such a spectacular end to my Olympic dream just devastated me. It seemed my whole world had come crashing down. I didn't know why, but knew I'd have to find out.

The phone rang again and it was David Knight. David now lived with his family in Hong Kong but had returned to Australia especially to watch me race. 'Come on, mate, grab your gear, we're going out,' he said. We went to a bar at Darling Harbour and talked about a lot of things, including the race. David is such a positive person to be around and was not about to let me sink deep into the trough of self-reflection. He reiterated what Jenni said, encouraging me to look at the good side—at least I made it to the Olympic Games. The general mood throughout Sydney was so upbeat it was hard to be too down. I had a few drinks, a few laughs and marvelled again at how lucky I was to have such great friends.

Penrith had been a refuge for most of my life. I felt very comfortable going home that night and was touched by the number of messages left on my voicemail by a whole range of people—family, friends and acquaintances from all over the world. Some offered congratulations for making the Olympics, some commiserated and some didn't know quite what to say so they just sent their love and best wishes. I went to bed hoping that I'd wake up and find it was all a bad dream. But of course it wasn't. I had been wishing for the fairytale all my life, but I was starting to realise that just wasn't my story. For some reason my journey through life has always been bumpy. I've never got things right straight away, but I think I am a good example of why you should never give up. I have been knocked down a lot but I always get up and keep on going. And I think most people find hope in that.

I didn't have long to process what had happened before I was back in training. I had to focus on the Paralympics now, and while I wanted to do well, I was really struggling to feel upbeat. The Australian team went into camp at Wollongong as part of the final preparation for the competition, and I was part of it. I am not particularly self-conscious but it was difficult to ignore the comments as I wheeled by: 'That's the guy who crashed.' There was no malice in those comments. I'm sure everyone felt for me, but pity was not something I wanted. I'd already put myself through hell in two of the toughest endurance events in the world to be seen as equal as an athlete, and the last thing I wanted to be remembered for was crashing during the Olympics. I knew the memory would fade, but the publicity I had attracted seemed to have built up expectations of what I might be able to achieve at the Paralympics.

It was not to be. Our 4 × 400-metre relay team bombed in the heat; I made it through to the second round of the 1500 metres, but not to the semi-final; I finished in the middle of the field in the 10 000 metres; I came tenth in the marathon, which was a good effort but well below my expectations; and I crashed again during the semi-final of the 5000 metres and was disqualified. In hindsight I think I made a mistake competing in so many events. I was racing just about every day of the Games. While many wheelchair athletes do just that, I would have been better off concentrating on one, maybe two events, and honing my skills to perfection in those. I'm not saying I would have won them, but I think I would have performed better. An Australian coach made a comment along these lines to me later on, and I had to agree with him.

My Olympic and Paralympic campaigns had fallen flat—and so had I. I didn't know it at the time but my less than stellar results, or, more importantly, my reaction to them, would be the catalyst for some overdue soul searching that would change everything. It was time to look inside myself—but, like most things in my life, it wasn't going to happen easily.

CHAPTER TWELVE

THE VALUE OF BALANCE

*'Look at what the guy has achieved. He is a
superstar athlete and a superstar human being
in terms of the way he has touched people's lives
and what he's given back to the community'*
—PAUL APPLEBY, BUSINESS ASSOCIATE

I was disconsolate after the Sydney Paralympic Games. I went home to hide from the world and everyone in it, rather like a snail retreating into its shell. My family and friends thought my depressed mood was an understandable reaction to a disappointing few weeks, that all I needed was a little time and I'd bounce back. They had seen me recover from setbacks before. I didn't have the heart to tell them that this was different. I wasn't just flat, something else was happening to me. I was spiralling down with no parachute or safety net to break my fall. It was a new experience—and I have to say I was scared.

What triggered this emotional meltdown? I can only speculate that it was a confluence of events. I had trained so hard and invested so much of my identity into doing well at the Sydney

Olympics and Paralympics that when I crashed so spectacularly, when I failed to perform to my true ability, it hit me harder than it should have. I can see now that I was too narrow in my focus. Achieving sporting goals was how I measured my worth as a person, and now that hadn't worked out the way I hoped I started questioning myself. The animosity shown towards me by some members of the wheelchair racing fraternity contributed to my depression. I was accustomed to sharing my journey with positive people who wanted me to do well, people who were prepared to go to the ends of the earth to help me achieve my goals. The exclusion I had faced in the run-up to the Games had been both hurtful and shocking, in that I hadn't anticipated it.

My past had caught up with me too. I'd never connected with my birth mother and the fact that she was the one I yearned for most when I was in Switzerland spoke volumes about my emotional state. I was yearning for unconditional love, but it seemed I had successfully side-lined every relationship I had ever been in. I was starting to ask myself, 'Why is this?' Maybe I was attracting the wrong sort of person, or maybe I was the one who was afraid to commit. I had never grieved the loss of Avril, nor the accident that made me a paraplegic. I mean properly grieved, really feeling the pain and mourning the loss. My day of reckoning had come.

I see this now as clearly and simply as night follows day, but that wasn't how I saw it at the time. I was just soldiering on as I had learnt to do as a child. ('Boys don't cry.') I was confused and despondent, and I didn't know how to dig myself out of this state of mind, or why I felt this way.

During this tumultuous period I was awarded an Order of Australia Medal for service to sport and the promotion and encouragement of junior wheelchair athletes, a big honour. Mum and Dad drove up from Culburra to share the occasion. They were so proud of me, and loved the ceremony at Government House where I received the medal from the then Governor of New South Wales, Gordon Samuels. I enjoyed it too, but the lift in mood was fleeting. I plummeted down again immediately afterwards.

I knew something had to change. I turned to Wally Brumniach, who'd been one of my support swimmers for the Channel. Wally was a straight shooter and I valued his opinion greatly. I rang him and said, 'Mate, I just don't feel very comfortable and it would be good to have a talk to someone.' Wally had often mentioned a guy he worked with, Maurie Rayner, a former AFL coach whom he fondly called 'Moses'. Maurie was a life coach who ran a centre in Victoria helping people confront their fears and ultimately live a more productive, meaningful life. He took executives on team-building exercises that exposed their vulnerabilities and encouraged them to face and overcome them. Among other apparatus he used a high-ropes course—ropes stretched between high poles with climbing harnesses and safety wires—as a fear-facing exercise. Maurie directed his clients to go out on the rope and move from one pole to another. Some of them would say, 'Great, let's go,' others felt fear and sometimes panic. Maurie would say to them, 'I am here for you. I will stay here until you conquer this.'

Wally said he'd call Maurie and see whether we could have a chat. Maurie agreed to see me—and this was a huge gesture, because he was dying of bone cancer. He had only a short time to live, but he invited me up to his Pottsville home in northern New South Wales to stay for the weekend. I don't know why he was so generous or giving with me, especially since we'd never met. But I am eternally grateful he was. Maurie became the master and I the student and he was able to say things to me that no one else could. Fortunately I was in the right space to receive it and learn from him. 'I'm dying and I'm incapable of bullshit, so let's get on with it,' he said when I arrived.

I told Maurie everything about my life—my early years in the children's home and Avril's illness and subsequent suicide, growing up in Tregear, the accident and my time in hospital, my failed sporting goals, my failed first marriage, my sporting successes and, of course, the Olympic and Paralympic Games disappointments which triggered the meltdown.

At the end of this story Maurie looked at me and said something I never expected to hear: 'The best thing that ever happened to you was getting hit by that truck.' To say I did a double-take would be a complete understatement—I was floored. But Maurie wasn't finished with me yet. 'The next best thing that ever happened to you was crashing at the Olympics,' he said. 'Maybe that will make you realise that life doesn't revolve around John Maclean.'

It had not occurred to me that I might need to go back before I could move forward.

By now Maurie had my undivided attention. He proceeded to tell me some more home truths—how my feverish goal-setting was getting in the way of my development as a person, how the answers I was seeking in life were not to be found in Hawaii or the English Channel or Homebush. They lay within me. He told me I didn't love myself, and that meant I was finding it difficult to let anyone else love me, especially women, whom I had to admit I had kept at arm's length for most of my life. He talked about Avril and the profound effect her death had on me. I had loved her, he said, and she had abandoned me, which closed my heart to other women. He said the core of my pain was my mother's illness and death, that processing and grieving that loss was critical for my recovery. I told Maurie about the challenges Dad had faced raising three young children, about his remarriage, how my step-mum hadn't grown up with affection and found it hard to show love. Maurie listened but laid no blame. 'You know your parents do the best they can do,' he said.

I listened intently to what Maurie had to say. He was giving me another perspective on my life. It was as if I was looking at myself from a completely different angle. No one would ever wish on anyone what had happened to me on the M4—that wasn't what Maurie meant when he said being hit by the truck was the best thing that ever happened to me. He was alluding to the fact that it had altered the course of my life. Before the accident I was a confident young footballer who hadn't thought much about the outside world or his true feelings or the meaning of life. I had no reason to be self-reflective because I felt I was a master of the universe. Maybe I could have resurrected my rugby league career after the blow-up at Penrith Panthers and gone on to play first grade—but if that had happened life could very easily have passed me by in a whirl. I'd never have become self-reflective, never travelled the path that led me to Maurie and the real soul-searching I needed to do to move forward in my life and find what I really wanted—love and happiness. The sporting goals I'd set to aid my recovery now completely defined who I was, at least as far as I was concerned. Crashing at the Olympics and Paralympics had been a wake-up call. I had to confront the big issues, including my feelings about Avril and why my exclusion at the hands of some of the Paralympians had been so hurtful. Maurie made it clear that at this point I was being presented with an important opportunity to find greater meaning and fulfilment in my life that was not to be squandered.

Maurie believed all people are born with pure love in their hearts. We start collecting what he called 'yuck bits'—unpleasant experiences—early on and file them away in our heads. 'As you get older those little yuck bits add up and it's my job to help you dissolve them,' he told me. 'By talking about what causes you discomfort, having the conversations around what the pain is, sitting with it for a while, understanding it, processing it and dissolving it, you are freer and more open to the whole love experience.' That was his message—face your fears and you conquer your demons. I had never thought about life like that. It had not occurred to me that I might need to go back before I could move forward.

The things we are told as children and how we interpret them are like the barnacles that attach themselves to a boat. The boat has a clean hull when it first goes in the water but it soon enough gets marked. When I was young, Dad, like most dads, would say, 'Boys don't cry. Stop your blubbing.' The more often you were told that, the more clearly you understood you were not meant to show emotion. From Maurie I learnt that it's okay to cry. He said, 'There are only two true emotions in life—love and fear.' His daughter lived not far away, and he told me that when his grand-daughter came to his house the first thing he always said to her was, 'I love you.' And, he said, '[Because she knows that] it doesn't matter what happens in her life, John, she'll be fine.' That showed me how strongly he believed in the power of the word 'love' and the connectedness it gives people in their daily lives.

I spent the weekend with Maurie and his wife Gwen, with Maurie giving me as much time as he could. It was a life-changing experience, and afterwards I understood the importance of having mentors who can help you along the way. Maurie was what I call a 'spirit tickler' (in other words, a 'spirit whisperer' who intuitively understands the real issues at the core of a person's troubles), and I'm so glad our paths crossed at that time. Years later Wally told me that Maurie had helped a lot of people achieve their goals in life. 'He was an expert at cutting through bullshit. I think he made you realise, John, that part of you was an act.' Sport was how I expressed myself but it was not all I was. I had more to offer, and I realised it was time I started concentrating on that too.

Maurie taught me that I was capable of having the life I dreamed of. What I needed was clarity around what that was. He asked me straight out, 'What *do* you want, John?' I told him I wanted a loving relationship. 'Don't be vague, be specific,' he responded. 'Is it a blonde lady, is it a brunette, a redhead?' What he was alluding to, which is the way I think now, is that you attract what you want. You can have the relationship you want. If you don't think much of yourself, if you just breeze along saying, 'Whatever comes my way is okay', that's what will happen. If you say, 'I would like to have XYZ lifestyle', you can attain it.

Maurie told me a story about a guy who'd always wanted a particular sports car but couldn't yet afford it. One day he went to the dealership, took a photo of the car and had it printed on a T-shirt, so that every time he wore it he would be reminded of his goal. Eventually he got the car. 'Be specific about what it is that you want,' Maurie told me. 'Eventually you may realise it's not what you thought you wanted after all, but it's one step at a time.'

He also told me about Albert Nobel, the Swedish chemist and industrialist who made his fortune from inventing dynamite. When he died in 1895 Nobel left most of his fortune to the establishment of a prize that celebrated the people and ideas that benefited and progressed humankind. Nobel himself had believed that dynamite would advance the cause of peace when people realised how armies could be utterly destroyed by it. By the end of his life, though, he realised he was wrong. He did not want to be remembered as the 'Merchant of Death' (which was how one French newspaper had described him in a premature obituary), but for good deeds, hence his bequest. The Nobel Prize is still widely regarded as the highest honour in the world in the fields of physics, chemistry, literature, peace, medicine and economics.

Maurie recounted this story to impress on me the value of giving back in life, or of paying good deeds forward so that their impact has a compounding effect. I couldn't help but wonder how I would be remembered. And, just as importantly, how did I *want* to be remembered? Surprisingly, it was not simply as the guy in a wheelchair who swam the English Channel and did the Hawaii Ironman. I realised I wanted to make a contribution, to give people—kids in particular—inspiration, to make them understand that regardless of the cards life had dealt them they could still achieve their dreams. I started thinking for the first time how I could best make a lasting contribution.

Maurie planted a seed in my mind, and I realise now how important it was. He shook me out of my malaise by challenging the way I looked at life, and what I was doing with my life. I learnt from him the value of balance. It wasn't healthy to concentrate all my energy on sporting achievements at the expense of developing fulfilling and meaningful relationships.

I went home with a lot to think about. I had changed. Not dramatically, but enough for me to realise things were not going to be the same again. It was as if I had reached a crossroads in my life and had paused to make sure I didn't take a wrong turn. This time I didn't set myself another sporting challenge and throw myself headfirst into it—I sat back. Maurie had found the key to my hidden reservoir of emotion, and it was time to let it all come out.

I started visiting my favourite locations around Sydney. I drove to the coast and spent hours looking out to sea. I went to the Blue Mountains and spent days watching the clouds and how the sunlight danced across the gum trees. The strong connection I've always felt with nature seemed to draw out my feelings like poison from a wound. I tried not to let my mind race, as it so often does, flitting instantaneously from one idea to the next. Instead I thought about the episodes in my life that had caused the greatest pain, and for the first time I didn't push them quickly to the back of my mind. I sat with them. When the tears finally came, I wondered if they would ever stop. I cried and cried and then I cried some more. I thought about Avril and felt the pain of the child who had never experienced that pure, precious love a mother feels for her son. I thought about living in the children's home and my lack of emotional security. I thought about the accident, about what it had cost me, about how much I still wished I could run. I thought about Michelle and mourned the end of our marriage—and the way I'd handled it so badly. I cried for all the sad times in my life and I cried for the good times. I thought of Johnno and how much he's done for me, and the tears came again. I went to the movies on my own, and if the movie was sad, I cried again.

This went on for some months. It wasn't a maudlin experience, though; more a purging of the pent-up emotions that had started to sour within me. I'm not saying this period of reflection solved all my personal problems or cured my aching heart, but it was a start. I had stopped moving long enough to allow my feelings to come to the fore, and even I was surprised at their intensity.

Maurie died in 2001, not long after our weekend together. I felt that an enlightened soul had left us, and I felt sad for Gwen and the loss she must be experiencing. Maurie was a unique human being who helped people overcome fear and tap into love. He was the master—and the right man for me to connect with at that time in my life. It would not have been right for me to meet Maurie pre-Olympics. I wasn't ready then. After the crash was the right time to stick up my hand and ask for help.

After Maurie's death, I started thinking about putting into action what I had learnt, to help other people as he had helped me. That would be paying his message forward and I couldn't imagine a better way of using my time. It wasn't long before I realised the vehicle for doing this already existed. The John Maclean Foundation, launched in 1998 after Nike gave me $20,000 for the charity of my choice, had been run under the auspices of the New South Wales Wheelchair Sports Association (NSWWSA) ever since. My initial aim was each year to help one boy and one girl aged under eighteen who couldn't raise the money to buy the equipment they needed to compete in their chosen sport. The NSWWSA identified the recipients and I presented the cheques at a yearly award night. The difference this made to people's lives cannot be overestimated. Money is so often an issue for families with physically challenged children. With no means of acquiring the equipment they needed—usually a specially designed wheelchair that enabled the child to play basketball or tennis or do athletics—many children missed out. The presentation of the cheques was something I looked forward to because I loved connecting with the families and seeing the joy on the kids' faces.

I had raised money through fundraising activities such as trivia nights, and the fact I worked with a range of sponsors also helped me connect people to the foundation. For example, I did a presentation along with some other athletes for Mercedes-Benz, and part of the deal was that we'd all get a car to drive for twelve months. However, Holden was sponsoring me at the time, so Mercedes-Benz gave me a van for the foundation instead. I put a logo down the side of the vehicle and then gave it to NSWWSA to transport kids in wheelchairs to camps and sporting events.

However, my involvement with the foundation was otherwise quite limited. After my experience with Maurie I started thinking seriously about making it more of a priority and taking the foundation to a national level. Money and exposure were the key issues. My first idea was to hand-cycle around Australia. I spoke to ultra-distance runner Pat Farmer, who'd 'circumnavigated' the country on foot in 1999. Pat cautioned me against such a venture, arguing—quite sensibly—that I would spend a lot of time traversing vast areas where no one lived. Not only would I raise no money in such places, I would attract limited publicity. He also warned of the dangers on some of the outback roads—particularly the road trains that used them as speedways. Did I really want to be negotiating such behemoths on narrow, often unsealed roads, choking in the dust and gravel they threw up? This made a lot of sense, so I revised my plans to a more modest but still ambitious trip down the east coast from Brisbane to Melbourne. I'd hand-cycle 2002 kilometres in 2002 and call the venture 'Kilometres for Kids' or 'K4K'.

Trips like this require a lot of organisation and behind-the-scenes work so I put together a team to manage the logistics. Steve Plakotaris (a friend of David Knight's) became the foundation's executive director and Trent Taylor, who had worked with the NSWWSA, agreed to be road manager. Years earlier I had asked a dear friend of mine, Alex Hamill, a former chairman of advertising giant George Patterson Bates, to be the foundation's chairman, and he'd kindly agreed. When I consulted Alex on the K4K concept he not only gave it his seal of approval, he made some calls and organised office space for us in North Sydney. Steve organised staff whose job it was to notify all the councils along the way, and the local media. We did a couple of reconnaissance trips and I met with police, mayors and a lot of previous sponsors. The support was overwhelming. We went to see Qantas and the people I dealt with there said, 'John, whatever you need.' That meant we had flights to destinations along the eastern seaboard when required. I spoke to Mercedes-Benz about vehicles and they said, 'Not a problem.' I rang contacts like Tony Garnett and he helped organise fuel, and my relationship with the Accor

Group saw our accommodation sorted out. The generosity of corporate Australia was heart-warming. I felt I was working on a huge jigsaw puzzle, but instead of cardboard pieces coming together it was human beings and what they could contribute to the picture.

As the task of organising K4K picked up speed, out of the blue I received a phone call offering me a spot crewing on a boat sailing in the 2001 Sydney to Hobart yacht race. The offer came from the computer company Aspect. Its boat competed under that name, but its slogan was 'Sailors With disAbilities'. I've always been uncomfortable associating myself with the word 'disability', but this was a great opportunity and I didn't want to pass it up. Skipper David Pescud took me for a test run through the Heads to see whether I was sailor material. Despite heavy conditions and rough seas I didn't turn green, so when we returned to dry land we discussed my role on the boat. I had made it clear I wanted to be actively involved or I wouldn't participate, so I was given the job of grinder, providing the muscle power to trim the mainsail. Modifications were made to the boat so my wheelchair could be anchored on deck and I trained with the crew on night runs up the coast north of Sydney—which I really enjoyed. It gave me a different connection to nature and an appreciation for the solitude of the sea.

As always, the Sydney–Hobart fleet set off on Boxing Day. Conditions in 2001 were relatively kind, but that doesn't mean we didn't get a taste of the power and fury of Bass Strait. At times the boat lurched at what seemed like right angles into the water but skipper and crew were experienced and capable. It took us about four days to get to Hobart and while I loved the experience I was pleased to dock and get back to a dry, warm, stable bed.

Back in Sydney, preparing for K4K became my main focus. The event was scheduled to begin on 1 June 2002. The goal was to finish the ride in thirty days, which meant we (the road crew and I) had to cover about 70 kilometres a day on average. With rest days factored in, we could be clocking as many as 140 kilometres a day; still a comfortable distance on the flat, but much more challenging in hilly country. A lot of my friends wanted to be involved and planned to do stages of the trip with me, either riding their bicycles alongside me or manning one of the support vehicles.

I never questioned my ability to make the distance, but I was experienced enough to enlist a masseur so I could get daily massages, especially on my shoulders. Taking Ross 'Rosco' Hutchinson along was one of my better moves, proving I had learnt something over the years.

I was always clear about the purpose of our trip—to raise as much money as we possibly could and create a national profile for the foundation. What I didn't fully appreciate before we set off was how personally inspired I'd be by the stories of kids in wheelchairs we met along the way. I thought I'd be a role model for them—but they became role models for me. We don't have to look far for amazing examples of courage and resilience; they can be found every day in homes and communities all over Australia.

One of my favourite stories concerns a boy named Jacob Ray. Jacob, whose paraplegia was caused by neuroblastoma, a type of cancer, lived in Culburra—where Dad and Mum moved after their retirement—and was the only kid in a wheelchair at his school. I was delighted when he contacted me in the lead-up to the K4K and told me of his plan to swim the Shoalhaven River to raise money for the cancer charity Camp Quality and the John Maclean Foundation. He was just eleven years old at the time. In March I went to watch him swim the Shoalhaven River, flanked by his swim coach and his local MP, and was doubly impressed when I learnt that he had raised $10 000. I dedicated the first kilometre of the K4K to Jacob Ray.

On 1 June the K4K started in Brisbane as scheduled. I had three support vehicles, one travelling in front of my hand-cycle and two behind. Our daily routine was meticulously mapped out. I got out of bed about 5.45 am, did any requested radio and press interviews, and hit the road early, trying to chew up the kilometres as quickly as possible. When we were approaching a town, we'd stop so Rosco could give me a massage, and I'd transfer into my wheelchair. We'd be met by kids from the town in their wheelchairs and we'd cover the last 100 metres together, to end the day pushing through a finishing chute organised by the crew. Most of the time the kids' families and friends, and many other locals, lined the roadside. Sometimes there would be hundreds of people clapping, cheering, and urging us on.

I loved this time spent connecting with the children, feeling their pride as they pushed their wheelchairs through town to rapturous applause. When I noticed that a lot of kids had far greater issues than not being able to afford sporting equipment, it got me thinking about where we were devoting our resources. If they were playing sport at least they were involved and getting out and about, but some kids rarely made it out their front door. It was then that I decided the reach of the foundation should be broadened to include non-sporting applicants. If we could provide a wheelchair to help kids engage in life in any way, that was as worthwhile as enabling others to play basketball or tennis. In the end we decided not to limit ourselves to providing wheelchairs—we have helped kids who want to play an instrument, and provided computers for better learning opportunities.

This was an important turning point for the foundation, a direct result of our trip down the eastern seaboard. Meeting the kids and seeing firsthand the problems they were facing on a daily basis made us want to help in any way we could. I was incredibly proud of this shift in focus, because the foundation has gone on to help so many kids in wheelchairs who originally didn't fit our criteria. I couldn't help but think of Maurie and his words of wisdom about finding balance in life and the joy of giving back to the community. I derived more joy from the looks on the faces of all the kids we met and helped and encouraged along the way than I had from just about anything else in my life and I felt very different, as if a void had been filled. I think it's what many people called contentment.

Surrounded by kids in wheelchairs and most of the other local school kids, we'd head to the town hall or shire offices to meet the mayor and other dignitaries. The local media was usually on hand and we'd do some interviews and take photographs with the kids. There was always a cup of tea and scones or cake to follow, and it was great meeting all the people who made the time to attend these civic receptions. Then we'd check into our accommodation. First off I'd soak in a hot bath to soothe my aching joints, then we'd hit the pubs and clubs and 'kick the can'. That meant carrying a bucket and talking about how we were riding from Brisbane to Melbourne raising money for kids in wheelchairs. We did this in every town we stopped in, and it was more tiring than the daily bike ride. If ever I had wanted an apprenticeship in how to engage and communicate with people, this was it. At the end of the night we'd count the money so it could be banked the next morning, then collapse into bed and prepare to do it all again.

Often I'd be invited to speak to a Rotary group or Lions Club meeting. I never knocked back these opportunities to promote the foundation and what we were trying to achieve with K4K. These networks are expert fundraising machines and many of them supported our efforts, for which I was truly grateful.

There was a great sense of camaraderie on the trip and many of the foundation's board members, like Alex Hamill, did stints with the crew, as did Dad and Johnno. Trent was the only person, however, who completed the entire journey with me. We developed a strong friendship and he went on to manage the foundation. Being on the road reminded me how much I liked being in a supportive team working towards a common goal.

I also learnt that the little boy inside me was alive and well. I've always had a penchant for testing the limits to anything I took on, and seeing how fast my hand-cycle could go was no different. On the NSW north coast I decided to find out, on a downhill stretch of the Pacific Highway outside Taree. I was travelling close to the lead vehicle with my favourite blues music blaring out at me. Being so close created a drafting effect—no wind resistance—and I was moving along at a greater speed than usual. This was my chance to go full throttle, and I opened up my shoulders and went for it. David Wells was driving, and had to accelerate to stay ahead of me as I notched 100 kilometres per hour. That speed on a hand-cycle is significantly fast and I could tell by the worried looks that my crew thought I had gone too far. Alex in particular was concerned, yelling at me at the top of his lungs, 'It's time to slow down!'

They were right, of course. But a few days later, between Bulahdelah and Newcastle, again on a downhill stretch, I felt myself gathering momentum. Again I went for it. Luckily I had only reached about 60 kilometres an hour when the hand-cycle's rear axle snapped and it veered wildly to the left. I struggled to keep upright, but the hand-cycle toppled, sending me skidding along the road, grazing much of my left side. It was a very lucky escape. If it had veered right, not left, I would have been thrown into the path of oncoming traffic and most likely killed instantly. Fortunately for me, David Wells is an ambulance officer, and he quickly patched me up. I was acutely aware of the mood of the crew and how concerned they all were—at what *had* happened, and what *could have* happened. Imagine the consequences if I'd been badly injured or, worse, killed? We cranked out the spare hand-cycle for the rest of the ride into Newcastle. After meeting the mayor and kicking the can around town, I went to bed that night very stiff and sore. I was paying the price for my crash—but it could have been a whole lot worse.

I enjoyed the great sense of community spirit I experienced in the towns along the route, but hand-cycling into Sydney and having a police escort across the Harbour Bridge was a real highlight. That sort of entrée is not afforded many people and I was determined to appreciate every minute of it. Dad was with me for that stage of the ride and I know he was blown away too. A lane of George Street was closed so we had an easy path to the Town Hall, where the Deputy Lord Mayor met me on the steps.

Dad left us in Penrith and Johnno joined the crew for the trip on to Melbourne. I'd been looking forward to this immensely, because he is always such positive company. Compared to our adventures in the north of New South Wales this part of the ride was relatively drama-free. We took in Canberra along the way and were met by Prime Minister John Howard. The biggest obstacle as we ventured south was the weather. Even though I had swum the English Channel, I'm not a great cold-weather person and found the chilly mornings and biting winds hard to handle, especially as we approached Melbourne and the conditions turned icy. On the final run into the city on 30 June we stopped for a while, and I sat in the car to warm up. It was so cold that I was concerned about hypothermia. We had a police escort all of that last day coming into Melbourne—half a dozen motorcycles travelling ahead of us clearing traffic and holding the lights. On the way down Swanston Street about fifty kids in wheelchairs joined in for the final run to the Town Hall and the waiting Lord Mayor. Over the thirty days of the K4K we had raised about $400 000 for the foundation and given it a national profile in the process. As I rubbed my hands together at the finish line to warm them up you couldn't wipe the smile from my face.

Alex Hamill had asked me quite early on, 'How big do you want the foundation to be?' I was a little taken back. 'I want it to be big.' 'Do you understand what that means?' he said. 'Sure,' I replied. 'We raise more money and help more families.' Alex pointed out the business side of the equation. 'If you raise more money and it starts to get bigger then you need to have office space and if it gets bigger again you need more staff and you start to minimise the percentage that actually goes to the cause.' I guess every charitable organisation wrestles with this problem.

I can't predict what will happen in the future, but my life has become entwined with the foundation. It's an interesting situation, but we are, I believe, co-dependent. Obviously the foundation wouldn't exist without me driving donations and spearheading corporate fundraising drives, usually around sporting events such as team triathlons and regional bike rides. But I have found over the years, and especially since that first K4K, that my equilibrium is slightly askew if I don't work at raising money. I love the presentation days and seeing the looks on the kids' faces when they're given a new wheelchair or some much-needed modification to assist their lifestyle, but it's more than that. I think being involved in the foundation has given me the balance in my life that was so sadly lacking before the 2000 Olympics. Maurie was right when he said the world didn't revolve around John Maclean.

That said, the foundation helps me too. Call it karma, or whatever, but good deeds beget good deeds. I know this. It's like a circle of giving and receiving. The more I give back, the richer my own life becomes. I'm not talking about financial windfalls or winning lotto. But the foundation has opened doors for me in other ways. I have forged lasting and meaningful friendships from my involvement with it and experienced things that I otherwise never would have. It's a symbiotic relationship—and I can't ever imagine breaking that tie.

To illustrate the point, a great thing happened to me after the K4K. I heard that I was to be the first non-American and first wheelchair athlete to be inducted into the Ironman

Triathlon World Championship Hall of Fame. I was asked to return to Hawaii in October that year to accept the honour and see my name etched alongside the greats of the sport. The president of WTC at the time, Lew Friedland, had the privilege of selecting one person each year for the Hall of Fame, and he'd nominated me for 2002. He told me later, 'It wasn't a difficult choice, John. It was so logical. You just persevered. You are an extraordinary athlete. To do all of that—all of those miles—with just your upper body is almost unimaginable.' Lew's words meant more than I could possibly express. He went on to say he didn't do it purely because I had inspired wheelchair athletes or broken down barriers, although they were important contributing factors. 'You were an incredible inspiration to able-bodied people too who fear not being able to accomplish things.'

I don't believe in coincidences. I believe that things in life happen for a reason. The timing of my induction into the Ironman Hall of Fame seemed to complement the fund-raising work I had done through K4K. It was as if the two were inextricably linked. I was on top of the world. I felt good about the contribution I was making through the foundation and ecstatic at the honour that was being bestowed on me halfway around the world in the event that had effectively launched my career and provided the cornerstone for my later sporting triumphs.

I returned to Kona with David Knight to accept the honour. While there, I tracked down my Ironman mentor, legendary Australian triathlete Greg Welch. He'd already won the event, in 1994, and was a giant of the sport. I wanted to tell him that it should be him being inducted into the Hall of Fame, not me. He just smiled and said, 'Grab it with both hands. You deserve it. My time will come.' And it did, in 2005.

My induction was a special moment in my life. David Knight gave an introductory speech that brought the house down. 'I have not had a bad day since I met John Maclean,' he said. 'I am now an Ironman because of him and I thank him for it every day. In one way or another, we have all been faced with pain and challenges big and small. But John's message is simple. No matter what happens in life, no matter what, never ever, ever, ever give up!'

There was not much I could add. I was emotional when I took the stage, and tried to keep it simple. Any challenge worth overcoming is hard, I told the audience. 'You've just got to keep going until you get to the finish line.' That's what I'd done here seven years ago, and ultimately it transformed my life.

CHAPTER THIRTEEN

HUMILITY

'He is who he says he is. He does have a goodness that translates into how he lives his life. What you see is what you get'

—Amanda Maclean, wife

My earliest memory in life is carrying a cup of tea in to my birth mother, Avril, who was 'lying down' in her bedroom in the family home in Tregear. I was three years old at the time. I remember how quiet it was as I entered her room, but have no recollection or image of her or what she said to me, if anything. I don't know if I made the tea myself or was merely a messenger sent to deliver it. I don't recall putting it down on the bedside table or walking back out of the room or any other detail about that experience, other than sensing her presence in the bed. Perhaps the memory is unreliable, but it tells me that Avril was in a dark place for a long time—and I am sorry about that.

After my weekend with Maurie I visited Avril's gravesite at Pinegrove Memorial Park in Minchinbury in Sydney's west. Although I had been there before, this was the first time I'd gone with an open mind and an open heart and with a few personal words of my own to say.

Avril was cremated, and her plaque is located on the edge of a small pond with a bird fountain in the centre. The fact that her ashes were buried near water was comforting, probably because I have spent so much time in pools, oceans and rivers and find water so soothing. I'd never addressed a gravesite before, but felt it was time the words were finally spoken out loud. I was the only one in the cemetery and found it incredibly peaceful. 'I wish it was different,' I said softly. 'I wish you hadn't taken your own life and I had known your touch and smell. I wish you were around to pick me up and kiss my cheek when I fell over and scraped my knee in the street as a kid. I wish you were at the hospital after I had my accident. I wish you were here now.'

I like to think Avril took her own life as the ultimate sacrifice for us—that she couldn't properly care for three young kids and didn't want to be a burden to anyone any more, least of all Dad. Maybe she thought she was setting us free, which is a nice thought to have when you have no other.

I never knew her, but it was time to acknowledge that I missed her. I think every boy's first great love affair is with his mum, and I hadn't had that intimate connection with mine. I couldn't bring her back or erase my own early life lessons as a result of her absence, but it was important for me to go back and reflect on her, in order to go forward again.

When I was lying on the track after crashing before a stadium filled with people at the Sydney Olympic Games, a powerful sense of *déjà vu* had swept over me. I felt I'd already lived that moment. I started thinking afterwards that maybe our lives were all mapped out and we were just playing our parts. Was this the case with Avril? Was her purpose having three kids, one of whom was me? Was it my purpose to get hit by that truck and go on to live a different life and help kids in wheelchairs? I'm still pondering those questions and readily admit I don't have the answers. I don't know what lies ahead when we die but I do hope I get to meet Avril one day, somewhere.

The words inscribed on her plaque are, 'We loved you so'. I looked at them for a long time, listening to the running water and the wind rustling through the leaves in the trees, and I realised that Maurie was right when he said I needed more balance in my life.

The all-consuming sporting goals I had constantly set myself could not be the only things I worked on. I had to invest more in my business career, friendships and family relationships—and in myself. I had to finally board that car on the emotional roller-coaster known as love and be prepared to drop my façade—my invisible wall—long enough to allow someone special to take the seat alongside. I remembered my response when Maurie asked me what it was I wanted out of life. I didn't hesitate: 'A loving relationship.' I was surprised at how much I yearned to meet the right woman and, hopefully, one day, have a family with her.

I'm not saying that after meeting Maurie I stopped setting sporting challenges for myself. That will probably never happen. I'm a competitive person and sport is a big part of who I am and what I do. But I started tweaking my priorities, taking care not to neglect other aspects of life.

During this period of reflection I turned to people whose advice I trusted. One of them was Marc Robinson, who ran the Australian operation of an American health care company in Sydney. We'd met in 1999, when I had spoken to his senior managers. After the presentation Marc told me how much he'd enjoyed my talk, and asked me to come back again and present to the wider company. We had hit it off straight away and not long after that he invited me to his home for dinner to meet his wife and sons. I liked Marc, especially for his unswerving devotion to his family. I saw him as someone who had his priorities in place. 'I want what you have,' I told him during one of our long conversations. 'I want a woman I can adore every time I see her and I want children.'

Not long after I met Marc he returned to the United States for work, but we still see each other as often as possible and speak regularly on the phone. I went to New Jersey for his son's bar mitzvah, a true privilege. His family welcomed me into their homes and lives as warmly as you greet a visiting relative, and through all my soul-searching post-Olympics I drew solace from the fact that Marc was only ever a phone call away. It's said you can count your true friends on one hand. For me, Marc is one of those people.

After returning from my induction into the Ironman Triathlon World Championship Hall of Fame I concentrated on training for the World Hand-cycling Championships, which were held in Prague in August 2003. It was a great trip. I didn't bring home a medal but I loved the Czech Republic and the architecture and sense of history that encased the city. I couldn't help but think about whether I would ever have made it there if my life had panned out differently and I hadn't been cycling on the M4 that fateful day.

That same year I reminded David Knight—who was now living in Connecticut—of a goal he'd set himself just after I had succeeded in swimming the English Channel six years earlier.

David promised he would attempt a crossing himself when he turned forty, so on his thirty-ninth birthday I rang him up and asked, 'Are you in training yet?' He was—he hadn't forgotten about it. David was a strong swimmer with a heart as large as humanly possible and it was an honour to be asked to be a part of the support crew for him, along with his mates Liam and Pierre.

As men are prone to do, David wasted no time in upping the ante. His goal was to not only swim the Channel—he wanted to attempt a double crossing. 'Imagine, David Knight in the history books as the first Australian male swimmer to do that,' he told me laughingly. 'This is a *big* deal. Forget Des Renford.' (Renford made nineteen one-way crossings.) David has a self-deprecating sense of humour, but I could tell the thought of his name being etched alongside some of the great endurance swimmers in the world, including Renford, meant something special to him. It just so happened that my original goal in 1998 was a double crossing, but the appalling weather conditions that forced me out of the water during my first attempt scuttled that idea. I thought it entirely fitting that I could now be involved in helping make David's dream come true.

David was well placed. Connecticut was a great hub for Channel swimmers and he was able to hook up with a squad and train in similar conditions to the ones he would be facing in the old ditch. His preparation was thorough and when we met up in London in 2004 before heading to Dover he was filled with confidence. The weather conditions that year had been bad and there were fewer crossings than usual. We waited a week for a window of opportunity, hoping the gale-force winds lashing the coast would ease. The timing of a double crossing was particularly tricky because invariably the swimmer had to choose between better weather conditions on the way over or on the way back. It's hard enough to find a window of 10-plus hours of calm seas and sympathetic tides for one crossing, let alone 20-plus hours for two.

On the day, the weather conditions were pretty good—a bit bumpy in places but not too bad. It took David 13 hours and 4 minutes to cross the Channel, nine minutes longer than it took me, but on touching French soil he made a critical error. He got out of the water for a ten-minute food break. The air temperature was colder than the water temperature and by the time he got back in he was freezing. In hindsight we all agreed he would have been better getting out of the water, touching the high-water mark on shore, which you must do for your swim to be officially recognised, then getting back in the water to eat his soup. But he didn't, and we will never know exactly how much of a difference that made.

Before the start of his attempt David had laid down some ground rules for his support crew, which included our mate Reg Brickell, the skipper of the boat that supported my swim and was now doing the same for David. If he made it to France, David wanted us to make sure he swam back. 'Don't let me back in the boat,' he said. He knew it was unlikely he would ever return to try again. But he also told us, 'Bring me back alive. I don't want to die doing this.'

I knew that David was feeling the pain, but he was in good spirits as we turned the boat around and he started the long swim back to England. By now it was after 10 pm and pitch black. Not long into the swim the weather started to deteriorate. After seven hours in the water David had only covered seven miles. At one point he became separated from the boat and we were all concerned. He told me later he wasn't concentrating and let himself drift off. 'It would have been so easy to slip away,' he said. 'I was in pain, it was cold and I was miserable and alone. I was thinking about the scene in *Titanic* when Leonardo DiCaprio's character Jack Dawson slips peacefully into the deep. Then I woke up and thought, "Not smart". I snapped out of it and thought, "Swim to the lights", realising that it was about survival—life, family and friends—so I headed back to the boat.' We were all worried about his mental state and kept asking him his phone number. I was swimming with David when he reached twenty hours in the water, and before I resigned my shift we stopped briefly and I asked Reg how he was tracking. He had 19 miles to go and he was travelling at a speed of one mile an hour. The weather was still bad and there was no change in sight. David might have been disoriented and out of juice, but he still could do the maths. He realised it was over but in typical fashion immediately made a joke. 'Anyone for breakfast?' he asked.

Channel crossing attempts are physically and emotionally draining. After David's swim I came home and took a couple of months off training. The swimming I'd done with David had reconnected me with the ocean and I wanted my next sporting challenge to be water-based. Of course, I had something in mind—the Molokai Challenge.

Held every year in Hawaii, this event is recognised as the World Surf Ski and OC-1 (open canoe, one person) Championships and the honour of winning it is what every waterman covets. The 32.3 nautical mile (60 kilometre) race begins near the west end of the island of Molokai, crosses the Ka'iwi Channel—renowned as one of the world's roughest ocean channels—and finishes at KoKo Marina at Diamond Head on Oahu.

My dear friend David Wells—who had been with me as part of my support team in Hawaii in 1995 and was an experienced surf lifesaver—had always wanted to compete in the event, so we teamed up, and our double ski was approved by the organisers. We trained with one of the giants of this event, Australian paddler Dean Gardner, who had won the event an impressive nine times and in 2005 was attempting to make it ten (he came third).

Some things you can do, some things you can't. Knowing when to call it a day is important.

I was welcomed into the paddling fraternity and race organisers couldn't have been more supportive of my inclusion in the field. They organised media to publicise my involvement to give the sport a bigger profile and we used it to raise awareness for the foundation. I was the first wheelchair athlete to ever compete and it was a fantastic experience. What I learned competing in Molokai was that the waves break to create a swell and you need to go with that because a wave propels you along until you get the next break—this was called getting a run. Trying to catch those breaks in a double ski was more difficult than in a single, which meant we weren't as competitive, but the beautiful thing for me was being able to line up with all those other great athletes and sharing the race's finish line.

The Molokai Challenge was held in May in 2005—and it was one of the most enjoyable sporting events I'd been involved in. However, it was not the most significant thing that happened to me that year. Early in 2005 I met a woman called Amanda. We immediately hit it off. At the time we were both involved with other people, but we kept in touch, often accompanying each other to functions. An easy friendship developed. We shared similar values and interests and she was one of the few women I had ever been able to enjoy silence with. Neither of us felt the need to fill the space with forced conversation or chitchat and that was so relaxing. There was an attraction but we kept it at a platonic level for about three years, continuing to date other people.

Meanwhile, David Knight called me about doing another event together. Not content with having competed in the Hawaii Ironman in 1999, 2000, 2002 and 2003, in 2006 he suggested we do the Ultraman World Championships in Hawaii, again on the Big Island itself, an endurance event that defies sanity. Over three consecutive days competitors cover 515 kilometres. On the first day it's a 10-kilometre ocean swim, followed by a 145 kilometre bike ride; on the second day it's a 276-kilometre cross-country bike ride, and on the third it's an 84.4-kilometre run, the equivalent of a double marathon. Effectively, the Ultraman is three Ironmans in succession. It's an invitation-only event and just thirty-five people compete each year. The Ultraman makes honest people out of all athletes who put their hand up to tackle it. If you aren't well prepared—physically and mentally—you will be brought undone, if not on the first day or the second, then certainly on the third.

As I expected, the swim was straightforward enough. The distance was no great problem and I was the second athlete out of the water. However, not long into the first bike leg I realised just how tough the event was. The bike leg involves an 1800-metre climb to Namakani Paio Park in the Volcanoes National Park, making the hills near Kona look tame in comparison. On a bike the elevation is achievable because you generate the power with the full strength of the quad muscles in your legs, but on a hand-cycle it was another matter altogether, and I missed the cut-off time that first day. Organisers allowed me to continue the event the following day, which started from Volcanoes National Park and involved a 1200-metre climb, but I pulled out halfway due to the incline. I returned on the third day and completed the double marathon, but technically I didn't finish the event.

David, on the other hand, was in with a great chance. He'd completed the first two days and at the start of the third was confident of pulling it off. But he is the first to admit he didn't train hard enough for the event and with about 10 kilometres to go, he started to falter. By this time I had finished the double marathon and had doubled back so I could support David to the finish line. He was starting to look slightly disorientated and was stumbling and struggling to stay on his feet. 'It's just an event, it's not worth your health,' I told him when he appeared in genuine distress. It was an awkward situation for us all, including Trent Taylor and Alex Hamill, who were there as part of our support team and who were now almost holding David up so he could put one foot in front of another. With about 400 metres to go we asked a doctor friend of ours to take a look at David and assess him. By now, he could barely stay on his feet and his eyes were rolling back in his head.

We found out later that what really alarmed the doctor was the fact that David had not lost any weight during the day, an indication that his kidneys were failing. An ambulance was called immediately and David was rushed to hospital. He was very sick, and very lucky that it didn't turn out differently. To this day I still find footage of those final minutes before he was withdrawn from the event chilling to watch. David left the island in a wheelchair. He recovered, but his family, quite rightly, were upset and worried. I think he learnt a great deal about himself that day—and I learnt a valuable lesson too. Some things you can do, some things you can't. Knowing when to call it a day is important.

I was still seeing Amanda occasionally. I never wanted to jeopardise my friendship with her, which made me more cautious than usual about getting romantically involved, even though it was becoming clear to both of us that our relationship could move to another level. We were at a blues club with friends one night when Amanda slipped away to the bathroom. A good mate of mine, Hans, leant over the table and gave me some sage advice. 'This is the one, John,' he whispered. 'Don't let her get away.'

Amanda travels quite a bit for work and was heading off overseas again. I had been given a bottle of Dom Perignon and told her I would share it with her on her return. I invited her to Penrith on Melbourne Cup weekend in November 2007 and she offered to make dinner. Amanda knows how much I love food and she is a great cook. It was perfect. We listened to music and talked and drank the Dom Perignon, and at the end of the evening it seemed only natural when I leant in and kissed her.

The next day Amanda put into words exactly what I was thinking. 'I value our friendship, and we should keep that in mind as we see what happens from here,' she said. I think I knew then that it was going to work out between us, but my mind was made up a couple of months later after I returned home from a business trip to Beijing. I developed severe food poisoning and thankfully Amanda was there to look after me, especially during the night when at one stage I fell backwards out of my wheelchair and lost consciousness. You can tell a lot about a person by how they react during the bad times and Amanda's care and compassion spoke a thousand words.

From that moment I knew she was the one. I wanted to marry her, but I wanted to get the marriage proposal right. I always regretted that I hadn't done it properly with Michelle, and it was important to me that it be romantic and memorable, something we could both look back on in our old age with fond memories and a warm smile.

Some years earlier I had been left a sum of money by my grandparents in Scotland. My aunt, Avril's sister, had called with news of the inheritance. I was very appreciative but decided that instead of money I'd rather have a family keepsake. My uncle Colin was in the jewellery business in Scotland, so I asked him to use the money to source a beautiful diamond and make me an earring, which I could keep forever as a memento of my grandparents and my Scottish heritage. He did exactly that. A few months later a 1.1-carat princess-cut diamond set in platinum turned up. It was a really beautiful earring, but quite ostentatious, and I only wore it a couple of times.

Now I had the earring made into a ring and I asked Amanda to join me for a weekend away. I took her to the Kings Tableland in the Blue Mountains, another of my special places. There was no one there except the two of us, admiring the beautiful view across the mountains. We were sitting on a ledge when I turned to Amanda and said, 'Sweet, they say you know when you know and I know. Will you marry me?' She said yes straight away and as I opened the jewellery box with the ring inside her eyes filled with tears of happiness. After that we went to a resort in Katoomba where I had booked a suite. I had arranged for a chilled bottle of Dom Perignon to be waiting for us, and we had an amazing night celebrating our engagement.

I had finally got it right.

CHAPTER FOURTEEN

NEVER GIVING UP

*'I have seen people inspired to change their lives
after meeting with John so it's quite an emotional
and life-changing interaction and impact he has'*
—Paul Appleby, business associate

O n this day, 11 September 2008, under a cloudless blue
sky at the Shunyi Olympic Rowing-Canoeing Park in
*Beijing, China, I have one final sporting goal to tick off before
I announce my retirement. Before I give it all away I want a
Paralympic medal. Not bronze, not silver, but glittering gold.
I don't think I am asking too much. I know I am a good athlete.
I have paid my dues, I have been around the block, and this
is my time. What better way to go out? A gold medal equals
excellence. It means that you are the best in the world on that
given day at that given discipline. And even more so for me,
to win a gold medal will be the culmination of a career in
sport, the icing on the cake, the last piece of the jigsaw puzzle,
which will allow me to move forward with my life, content in
the knowledge that I was not only the best I could be but at
one stage, however briefly in time, the very best.*

When I was twelve, I won a gold medal in race-walking. Representing Nepean Little Athletics Association, I had qualified for the event by winning the district, zone and state championships. It was my third attempt. At ten, I was disqualified in the State Championships. At eleven I came third and at twelve I won the gold medal in the National Championships at Bruce Stadium in Canberra. Standing on the podium I looked around and thought, 'Cool!' It's thirty years since that happened.

It makes sense to me that winning a Paralympic gold medal is meant to be. Winning one means my sporting career has come full circle, and that seems a great way to go out. Since setting myself this goal I have gone to bed every night with a photocopied colour photograph of the gold medal stuck to the wall opposite my bed. I have another in my gym, another on the fridge and a fourth one on the wall facing me in my office. The philosophy behind this is: If I don't see it, how can I get it? If I merely think, 'Hey, it will be really cool to make the podium', it's likely I won't win the gold, I probably won't win the silver, although I might, just might, win a bronze. If I only think, 'How good would it be to be part of the final?', then I won't even make the podium.

When you are racing and it gets really hard—and it will get really hard—it is easy to let yourself think, 'Okay, I am comfortable with second or third' or 'I am comfortable with making the final' or 'I am comfortable with getting a tracksuit'. An athlete's mindset pivots on these points. That's why there can be no compromise, no room for doubt. The focus *must* be the gold medal because that is the best way to end my career— and I believe it will happen. For me right now, anything other than that is unacceptable, absolutely unacceptable.

I am a good athlete but I am not a natural rower like Australians Drew Ginn and Duncan Free, who won the Olympic gold medal in the men's pair in Beijing. They are not only born to the sport, but also to the boat. Tall and lean, with the strength and the tactical smarts to boot, they have the ability to be as one, moving back and forward in perfect unison to extract the maximum power in the most efficient way. They have spent years perfecting their sport, and they live and breathe it.

I've done a lot of kayaking over the years up and down the Nepean River with my best mate Johnno. We have paddled a few times in the 111-kilometre Hawkesbury Canoe Classic, coming close to winning our category one year. But rowing? No. It is as new to me as the marathon would be for Australia's 400-metre sprint champion Cathy Freeman or the 1500 metres would be for American swimming superstar Michael Phelps.

A gold medal equals excellence. It means that you are the best in the world on that given day at that given discipline.

Yet rowing was my event in Beijing. I took up the sport in February 2007, when Gary Foley, a wheelchair athlete coach I met in the lead-up to the Sydney Olympics, rang me out of the blue. I hadn't heard from him in ages. 'Have you heard of adaptive rowing?' he said. 'No,' I replied. Gary explained that rowing is the youngest sport in the Paralympic Games. It was introduced to the program in 2005 and the first Paralympic contests were to be at Beijing. Adaptive rowing means the equipment is adapted to the user to practise the sport, rather than the sport being adapted to the user. I needed a partner to compete, as simple as that. And it had to be a woman. These were the rules, and while I had never attempted any such feats before—rowing, rowing with a partner, rowing with a woman— they were challenges I was up for, absolutely.

'Well, what do you think?' Gary asked. I made the decision to try out on the spot. It would be an amazing opportunity to get another crack at what had eluded me so disappointingly in Sydney—a medal of any hue, but gold in particular.

Gary told me to go down to the Sydney International Regatta Centre in Penrith, just ten minutes from home, and meet the coach, a Swiss guy called Pedro Albisser. I did so the next day. Pedro said, 'I'll put you on a rowing machine and see if you can produce a result.' I needed to clock a time of less than 4 minutes 20 seconds for 1000 metres on the ergo machine or I wouldn't be considered. I went 4 minutes 10 seconds—and from that moment it was game on.

There were lots of things I needed to know about rowing, but there was only one question I wanted to ask: 'What do I need to do to win a gold medal?' I wasn't going to begin this process— and commit the time and energy required—unless I could be as sure as it was possible to be of the outcome. I was not going to put my life on hold for eighteen months and be strict about diet and training unless the realistic likelihood was gold. If I couldn't believe that, I wouldn't start.

'The first step is the State Championships next weekend,' Pedro said. 'Then you need to go to the Nationals in six weeks time—and if you win your category and if there is a girl who wins hers and your times are good enough you will go to the selection regatta and compete together. If you produce a good enough time together you make the Australian team, and you go to the World Rowing Championships in Munich later this year. If you make the final there, you qualify the boat for Beijing.'

Completely unprepared, I went to the State Championships to compete against four other rowers. I was last out of the blocks and going nowhere when a race official in the boat tailing the field began telling me to relax. My frustration must have been as obvious as my lack of speed. I gradually got into a rhythm of sorts and finished second, which was good enough to qualify for the National Championships. These were held at Nagambie, a town 120 kilometres north of Melbourne in Victoria, which sits on the shores of Lake Nagambie, a national standard rowing and canoeing course. It was windy and dusty and a day I don't remember in great detail, except for two things: it was the first time I would meet a young Victorian woman called Kathryn Ross, who would become my rowing partner in Beijing; the other thing was the protest from another competitor that almost derailed my medal dream before it had a chance to embed itself.

The officials had combined a couple of categories on this day, which meant that as a trunk-and-arms rower I was competing against some arms-only rowers. We were racing over 500 metres, not 1000 metres as initially planned. I was told I would have to pull a Velcro strap across my chest to level the playing field for the other competitors. I have the use of my lower back and some leverage from my legs, so the strap was designed to eliminate any advantage I might have over rowers whose physical challenges were more severe. I was a little concerned because I had never rowed with a strap on before, but Pedro told me not to worry about it and to loosen it a little once I was out on the course so I didn't cause myself an injury. The night before the race one of my fellow rowers was overheard dismissing my chances in the event. 'Maclean's no good,' this guy said. 'He doesn't have any speed.' The comment got back to me, and only served to sharpen my resolve. I got to the start line, loosened the strap as instructed and went on to win. Celebrations were short-lived, however, when a fellow competitor lodged a protest immediately after the race. 'You were supposed to have your strap up higher,' the official told me. 'Okay,' I said. 'I'm disappointed, but if that's what it is, that's what it is.'

No national medal, no qualification. But before I could begin to dwell on the real disappointment, the shattered Olympic dream, I was pulled aside by Adam Horner, the manager of the rowing team for Beijing, and introduced to 26-year-old Kathryn Ross. He wanted to put a two-person mixed crew together to compete against the Americans at the World Rowing Championships in Munich, who hadn't been beaten in this event in five years. He wanted Kathryn and me to be that crew.

Kathryn hails from Warrnambool in Victoria. At the age of two and a half she'd been knocked over by a ride-on mower on the family property, suffering severe leg injuries when it came back over the top of her. It was Father's Day. She was flown by air ambulance to the Royal Children's Hospital in Melbourne, where doctors were initially concerned about infection, but over the ensuing years faulty bone growth saw her in plaster and undergoing operation after operation. Kathryn loves swimming, but wasn't quite good enough to make the Paralympic team in that sport. As part of the Australian Paralympic Committee's talent identification program, she was urged to try rowing.

One of my favourite sayings is 'control the controllable'. In other words, focus on what you *can* do in life, not on what you can't. After my accident I could have made myself miserable by concentrating on the things I couldn't do—I couldn't run, I couldn't walk on a beach, I couldn't this, I couldn't that—or I could turn that around and say, 'I won't worry about that, because I have no control over it.' I knew from the start that there wasn't an opportunity to participate at the Paralympic Games in rowing on my own. This was a mixed doubles event, locked and loaded. Therefore, my view was, let's hope there is somebody else with an interest, let's hope she's competitive and let's go and have a crack. Kathryn and I both came to the sport wanting to be the best we could be. Her goal was making the Paralympics, mine was the gold medal.

'control the controllable'. Focus on what you *can* do in life, not on what you can't.

Being a part of any team is a huge challenge. Being a part of a team with male and female competitors is a different dynamic altogether. They say men are from Mars, women from Venus. Sometimes I'm surprised we're even in the same universe. Kathryn and I are opposites. She likes country and western music, I like André Bocelli; she watches *McLeod's Daughters* and has every episode on DVD, I like wildlife documentaries; she likes to wear make-up in the boat, I don't care whether I've shaved; she is Generation Y, I am Generation X.

The thing that we do share is what I call the giddy-up factor—when the going gets tough, we refuse to lie down. Kathryn had an accident when she was very young, was picked on at school and selected last for sporting teams by her peers, but she persisted with a fiery determination that I have grown to admire.

The Paralympics are her time to shine, and my dream for her is to go back home as Queen of Warrnambool. It's the first time I've partnered with a female athlete in a competition, let alone a competition on a global scale. But I won't say it's more difficult than any other challenge I've taken on. It's just different. In many ways it's brilliant because it's all about teamwork. Managing it is the key. I want us both to learn and grow from the experience. I hope I'll be able to take something out of it and apply it in a business context around teamwork, understanding people's strengths and weaknesses. Kathryn says that her biggest fear is of letting me down because it's my last throw of the dice. I say, 'It's not about me, Kat. It's about you. I don't wake up in the morning looking at you; you wake up in the morning looking at you. You live your own life. Don't worry about me. Start thinking about yourself.'

Adaptive rowing—more than any other sport I've been involved in—is about harmony. I went into it thinking that rowing was all about power. And while yes, that's critical, it's not the only component of a good rower. Kathryn and I need to be at one in the boat. It's like a double pendulum. I am at the bow, which means I sit behind her. The more I can mimic her—almost like a shadow—the faster we go. If I can place my blade at exactly the same time as she does, and exit it at the same time, and we can establish the rhythm that rowers talk about, then it's a beautiful thing. The boat just hums in the water and it feels fantastic. When the boat is not running that way you use more energy and it's a lot more painful. It's surprising how far 1000 metres can be when your blades are out of sync and you're not in time.

Kathryn sets the stroke rate. My strength is to produce as much power as possible to support her, all the while keeping in unison. I never talk to her during a race. At the 250-metre mark I am close to maximum heart rate, at 500 metres I am there, at 750 metres I am doing whatever I can to hold the rhythm—and by the end of the race, I'm shot. I can't talk because I am trying to breathe.

Any athlete will tell you the importance of a strong mental attitude. It's as critical to good performance as technique. Many talented athletes have had their dreams shattered by insecurities that either don't allow them to win or put obstacles in their path that trip them before the finish line. In team sports, encouragement is critical. Kathryn was no different. Growing up with her injuries affected her self-esteem. Being left out of team sports or being the last to be picked in the playground leaves an indelible mark on most people unlucky enough to go through that, and it did on Kathryn, definitely. My job was to bolster her. If one of her strokes wasn't clean in the water, I'd say, 'Forget about it. Get back in the stroke as quickly as possible.'

I call her my younger adopted sister and say, 'This is your time. This is not just about a gold medal, it's about a gold-medal life. You deserve a gold-medal relationship; you deserve a gold-medal job. You deserve gold medals throughout your whole life. Until you believe that, you are not going to get it.'

After the Nationals, Kathryn stayed with me in Penrith for ten days to practise with me for the selection regatta and familiarise herself with the facility that has become my second home over the years. This was where I started training for the English Channel swim. I haven't calculated the figures, but I think I have clocked more kilometres swimming the Penrith Lakes than many people have clocked in their cars.

Our intensive training paid off. We made the team at the selection regatta in April and recorded a good time. In May Kathryn fully relocated from Warrnambool so we could ramp up our training together. A few months later, in August, we set off to Munich for the 2007 World Rowing Championships, the last hurdle we had to clear before we were Beijing-bound. To qualify the boat we had to make the final in Munich. Unlike the Olympic Games and Paralympic Games, which are held at different times, the World Rowing Championships are inclusive. We were part of the Australian rowing team, which was fantastic. All athletes—able-bodied and physically challenged—competed in their respective categories on the same course at the same regatta. We loved it that we could connect with the other athletes.

I met three-time Olympic gold medallist Drew Ginn in Munich. I went up to his rowing partner Duncan Free—they look very much alike—and said, 'Hi Drew, my name's John.' Oops. He said, 'I'm Duncan, Drew's over there.' They are giants of the sport and in 2007 the International Federation of Rowing Associations named them the World Rowing Male Crew of the Year. Drew and Duncan watched us win a silver medal in Munich, coming second by a boat length to Brazil. Surprisingly, the five-time American champions dropped out of the medal placings, indicating just how tough the competition had become.

After the race I got a chance to talk to Drew. 'Did you notice anything that I could work on to improve?' I asked. Yes, he said, there were quite a few things, not surprising as I was so new to the sport. 'John, what you need to do is switch off your power. You're trying to use power all the time and you are not being efficient in the boat. It's a process of coming forward, placing the blade and being in control and relaxed with power.' Pedro always came back to us with details on techniques and blade work and it was helpful and encouraging that Drew had just re-emphasised this.

Once I set a goal, an important part of my strategy for achieving it is get expert advice and soak up as much knowledge as I can. I am not afraid to ask questions because I am the first to admit I don't have all the answers. Before I embarked on my preparation to swim the English Channel I went to see Des Renford, the man who had swum it nineteen times from nineteen attempts. Before the 2000 Sydney Olympics I had lunch with Herb Elliott, the world champion 1500-metre runner, who was never beaten in the event from 1958 until he retired in 1961 at the age of twenty-four. It was the same with rowing. After the Munich event, I took Drew Ginn to lunch in Melbourne and plied him with more questions. I was asking, asking, asking, trying to short-track the path to success.

Qualifying for the Beijing Paralympics is like ticking another box. Kathryn and I have a year to improve our technique and our race times, and our training regime has increased accordingly. As the countdown begins, we have one more international regatta to hone our skills and check out the competition. In April 2008 we travel to Gavirate in Italy for the International Adaptive Regatta. We win the gold medal, beating the Italians by one and a half boat lengths, with the English pair jagging third. Brazil doesn't compete. Despite the win, Pedro is annoyed with us for not keeping to the pre-arranged race plan, which was holding 36 strokes a minute to the finish line. Fair comment, I think.

The English team's third in this regatta was a wake-up call—they had improved their time significantly since the World Rowing Championships. When we found out they were training full time, courtesy of the UK lottery system that funds many athletes and their dreams for success, it was time for Kathryn to give up her job so we could train full time together. We discussed how much money she would need to make that possible, and then I set about trying to make it happen. I have been a professional athlete for more than a decade, but that doesn't necessarily mean I am paid by the sports or events I compete in. It's sponsorship and corporate work that pays my bills. Necessity—and the help of some generous and wise people along the way—has taught me how to build a business around my achievements, but I would be lying if I said there weren't times early on when I was struggling to make ends meet, when a can of baked beans was the only food in the house and I didn't know where the next pay cheque was coming from. Kathryn had some savings and her family pitched in. She received a grant from the Australian Sports Commission, and a local business agreed to contribute as well. My relationship with the mayor of Penrith at the time opened a door that allowed me to put forward a sponsorship proposal to a local business. They generously provided funding not only for Kathryn and me but also for Pedro and the Lakes Rowers.

The funding means that Kathryn can start training full time in May 2008, allowing her to concentrate her energy and focus more fully on the task at hand. We are training six days a week, sometimes three times a day, for up to five hours. Not only are we on the water, rowing as many as 12 kilometres per session, including fixed race pieces and practice starts, but we're doing strength and conditioning work at the NSW Institute of Sport at Homebush and using their heat chamber—set at 30° Celsius and 75 per cent humidity—to try to acclimatise to the conditions we will face in Beijing. We are hand-cycling twice a week, doing weights in my home gym, and recovery sessions too, to give our bodies the best chance of reaching their full potential.

Our event category is called mixed trunk and arms, 'mixed' meaning the same as in mixed doubles tennis, and 'trunk and arms' meaning we pivot from the pelvis, using our upper body, because we can't use our legs. Our boat is a lot wider than a conventional scull for stability and thus weighs a lot more, requiring a lot of effort to move it over the 1000-metre race distance. Our seats are fixed and not sliding, therefore our legs do not come into play, although we do try to brace off them to get a bit of extra leverage through the stroke. We have a strap above our knees and our feet are Velcroed into place. This is to provide as level a playing field as possible for all competitors, whose physical challenges vary enormously. For rowing, you need a strong lower back and good core strength, but after being in a wheelchair for twenty years my lower back is my weakest spot, other than my legs, so I do lots and lots of sit-ups and hyper-extensions to make my back as strong as it can be. We see a physiotherapist once a week, a massage therapist and a dietician, to make sure we are eating the right type of food to keep our weight down, and we are taking mineral and vitamin supplements with no contaminants that might show up in urine and blood tests. Through my sponsorship with Gatorade we are accessing sport science experts who do scientific sweat testing in a heat chamber. I sweat very heavily, and in analysing the sweat test results they are able to advise the level of replacement energy, hydration and sodium I required.

The final piece of our preparation was the race plan. At Munich we had started badly. We were last out of the blocks but still managed to mow down the rest of the field except Brazil, who gained five seconds on us in the first 50 metres. We pulled back two of those seconds over the course, but could not make up the rest. Our starts had improved dramatically since then.

Our plan for Beijing is to go about 42 strokes a minute for the first ten strokes, and then ease back to 36 strokes a minute. We also need to be really conscious of staying long. This means making sure we place the blade in the water before pulling back. When you think about it, this makes sense. Once the blade is in the water you can start what they call the body rock to pull with your arms and come back while the blade is engaged, rather than starting to go before it is in the water. When we drop our stroke rate down to 36, it gives us just enough time to come forward and recover before placing the blade again. The theory of rowing is that you apply the power on the way back and you recover on the way forward. So it's not like you are rushing to go forward as quickly as possible, because if you did that you would fall apart at the back end of the race.

Our personal best time for the 1000 metres is 4 minutes 9 seconds, and we did that by doing 36 strokes from the start. We know we can do better and the race plan we have come up with bears testament to that. We want to get moving quickly so that we can establish momentum. It's a standing start and you want to get your boat up to speed as fast as possible. If we miss the start, like we did in Munich, we will be working really hard to pull the other guys back—and that's very difficult to achieve. We want to go out with the others and quite possibly be a little bit ahead, but not to the extent of using too much energy in the first 250 or 500 metres. We want to make sure we can bring it home.

Our plan is to break the race into four even splits. We want to go 1 minute 2 seconds per 250 metres, which will give us a race time, depending on conditions—tailwind or headwind—of 4 minutes 8 seconds, which could give us a 3-second better time than Brazil's winning time at the World Championships.

It is going to be a tight race, but we know the Brazilians have their own challenges. It will be difficult for them to improve on their time given they are so explosive out of the blocks. At Munich Brazil came first, we came second and Poland came third, followed by Italy and the United States. At Gavirate we won the gold medal, Italy won the silver and England the bronze. China did not qualify their boat at Munich, but as the host nation I am sure they will be racing. But it's Brazil that's going to be our main competitor.

The rowing at Beijing was scheduled over three days. There were to be two heats on the first day, with six countries in each. The winners of each heat would qualify immediately for the final, and the other ten go through to the two five-boat repechages to be held the following day. The first two placegetters from each of the repechages would go through to the final.

I don't think they will put Brazil and Australia in the same heat, but if they do part of me is saying, 'Bring it on. We'll see them off to the repechages.' We aim to win our heat and go straight through to the final.

In the final it's going to be neck and neck with Brazil to the end. If we get our race in order we will be ahead at the 500 metre mark—and that's where it really starts to hurt—and the team that holds it together will cross the finish line first. At 750 metres Brazil are still going to be around but we are definitely capable of beating them.

That's what I see. Kathryn is seeing us pipping them at the post, but my dream is to do better than that. I think it's important psychologically for Kathryn to see herself with the gold medal. So two months before Beijing I take her to sit on the podium at the Sydney International Regatta Centre where the medals were presented to rowers during the 2000 Olympics and Paralympics. I say: 'Kathryn, I want you to visualise the people in the grandstand and the Australian flag and hear the national anthem.' We do it again a month later and one more time before we go. I'm trying to get Kathryn to see my vision. If she can see it, she will believe it, and she will achieve it.

We left Sydney with the Australian Paralympic Games team on board a specially chartered Qantas jet on Monday 1 September 2008, five days before the opening ceremony in Beijing. We'd all stayed the previous night at the Airport Ibis Hotel and the excitement was palpable. Media interest was high and Kathryn and I did a 6.30 am interview for Seven Network's *Sunrise* program on the day we flew out. My phone was running hot with messages of support and good wishes, as I am sure was true for all the athletes. I spoke to Steve Waugh, the former Australian cricket captain, whom I'd got to know a few years previously when he invited me to be part of a program he was running with schools called Chase Your Dreams. Steve had interviewed Olympic champion Cathy Freeman, surfing great Layne Beachley, singer Shannon Noll, cricketer Michael Clarke, tennis legend Pat Rafter, and me, about the events that shaped our lives, and in March 2005 a DVD of those interviews was distributed to all Australian schools. I also heard from Li Cunxin, better known as Mao's Last Dancer. Li grew up in Qingdao on the coast of north-east China, the sixth of seven sons in a poor rural family. At eleven, he was chosen by Madame Mao's cultural advisers to study dance and went on to become a principal dancer for the Houston Ballet. He defected to the West in 1981 and now lives in Melbourne. We have become good friends over the years.

The flight was uneventful but when we arrived in the Chinese capital in the late evening we knew we were somewhere different—and it wasn't only the humid conditions and the architectural marvel that is Beijing Capital International Airport that told us that. There were officials everywhere looking to assist. Our arrival ran like clockwork. There were armed guards at every turn and special traffic lanes set up for Olympic vehicles. The Olympic Village was a first-class facility. The next morning we had a group meeting with the Australian Paralympic Committee and members of the Australian Federal Police, who talked about the difference in culture and what we could expect. 'This is not Australia, this is China,' we were told. 'If you're seen to be promoting the Dalai Lama or anything in relation to political statements they will take you and put you in jail and then you will be deported. If you are seen to be excessively drunk or acting in a manner that's not seen fit, you will be arrested. This is not Australia and you need to abide by the laws of the land.'

I am in China for one reason, and one reason only: to win a gold medal. I'm not going to get caught up in politics or socialising or even going to the opening ceremony because I want to stay completely focused on what I am here to do. I don't want to distract myself a couple of days before our heat by doing anything that will break my concentration or sap my energy. Not like I did at the Sydney Olympics.

I didn't want to make the same mistakes by getting caught up in the moment, eating the wrong foods, socialising and enjoying the ceremony and participation with leading athletes. The Opening Ceremony in Sydney was a memorable experience, but it took my focus off my main goal.

Life in the village was as relaxed as it could be before such a big event. In the mornings I did a urine sample which was analysed to see if I had dehydrated in the warm, humid conditions, had breakfast, and then booked a massage or some time with the physiotherapist. I'd hang out watching DVDs, or listening to music on my iPod and reading and sending emails. After lunch the rowing team was bussed out to the Shunyi Olympic Rowing-Canoeing Park about fifty minutes away for a practice session, which Kathryn and I scheduled for the same time each afternoon as our race. When we got back in the late afternoon I would have an ice bath. This is a cold water bath with added ice bringing the temperature down to around 15° Celsius; the cold helps flush lactic acid from your muscles and eases muscle fatigue.

The draw for the two heats in our event comes out the night before. Kathryn and I feel the draw for our heat is a pretty good scenario. We haven't drawn Brazil, Italy or Great Britain—we've got the United States, China, Ukraine, Germany and Canada. We think the United States will be our main opposition; we are conscious that China is in our heat too, although we don't see them as a threat—we've never seen them race.

The adrenalin and excitement were building. We woke the next morning to a cool and rainy day. I was trying to stay as relaxed as possible to save all my energy for the race. Our heat was scheduled for 4.20 pm so we left the village around 1 o'clock to ensure plenty of time for getting to the course and beginning the final stage of our preparation. Beijing traffic is notoriously heavy, but during both the Olympics and the Paralympics half the city's cars were taken off the roads.

We immediately make our way to the boat shed, which has a clear view down the course. There are a few gym mats lying around so I do some stretching to pass the time and to get off my backside, which gets painfully sore if I sit for too long. This is where I start to feel really nervous. My heart rate rises considerably and I'm sure so does my blood pressure. Kathryn and I change into our zooties—close-fitting rowing suits—and head off to the pontoon to get our final words from Pedro. We get into the boat, which we've named Only Possibilities, *in recognition that positive thoughts produce positive results. We move up the left side of the course, the warm-up area. We do a few 20-stroke and 5-stroke race pieces and a practice start. We feel pretty comfortable, just like we do on our home course at Penrith.*

With about ten minutes to go, we are called to the start line and row under the bridge onto the course proper. We are in lane 5, and at this stage I'm thinking, 'Let's go. Let's get on with it.' We move into our lane and a little gate like a Perspex cone comes up out of the water; this is where the nose of the boat sits. I tell Kathryn to have a quick look down at the course, so she can get a feel for the conditions. There's a pretty strong headwind, so I say, 'Remember, tap down at the back end', which means 'really push right down to clear your blade from the water'. An official asks, 'Australia, do you want us to check your boat?' We nod and a guy jumps into the water and checks under the fin for weed. Now we're in the starter's hands. 'Attention, please!' he says in English. And we wait, and wait, and the siren sounds. He drops the gate and we're off.

I could sense that the other boats got off really quickly. We didn't. We had a dreadful start. At the 250-metre mark we were in clear second place, but 2.34 seconds behind China. At the 500 mark we had fallen further back, and were now 4.43 seconds behind. We were still clearly in second place, but that was no consolation. Only the winner made it straight through to the final and earned a rest day, so if we wanted to stay true to our race plan we needed to pull something extraordinary out of the hat—and hope that China had gone out too hard to maintain momentum at the back end of the race.

We are starting to find our rhythm. At the 750-metre mark, we've pulled back China's lead to 4.12 seconds and we're gaining on them. But it isn't enough. At the finish line we come second by 3.99 seconds, or more than a boat length. China has never been on our radar and has surprised us, and the adaptive rowing world, with a comprehensive and unexpected victory over one of the event's favourites.

I'd be lying if said I wasn't a bit shocked and disappointed by the result. So was Kathryn. Neither of us was in a position to know immediately what had happened, but we found out later that China's technique, while not textbook perfect, was effective because their stroke rate was unusually high—about 55 strokes a minute. They'd set their boat up a bit differently too, with not as much resistance on the gates that hold the oars. And they weighed less than we did, so they could afford to rate higher.

We got on the bus and went back to the village. We'd had a shocker, but the way I looked at it, better in the heat than in the final, because you can't turn the clock back then. Kathryn and I wrote down what had gone wrong and what we needed to do to reverse the result the next day. Sometimes you can hear something, sometimes you can see it, but if you write it down it somehow makes it clearer.

We woke to sunny skies on the morning of the repechage. Gone were the grey clouds and misting showers. It was as if the sun was sending us a message. The mood was different, too. I was just as nervous at race time, knowing that more was at stake because it was now about qualification or elimination, but somehow it felt better. We were in repechage 1, racing Great Britain and the United States, Israel and Canada. Only two of us would go through to the final, but we had beaten both Great Britain and the United States previously and I knew that gave Kathryn a boost in confidence.

It's another headwind, but we start strongly and pull away from the field straight away. At the 250-metre mark we are almost 3 seconds in front of the United States, with Great Britain third. We extend our lead throughout the race to record a time of 4 minutes 31 seconds, almost 11 seconds in front of second placegetters Great Britain and 40 seconds in front of the United States, who come in third, ahead of Israel and Canada.

I felt relieved, as much as anything. We had rowed a smooth race, but not a blistering one. We'd done the job and made the final, and that's what we'd needed to do.

After the repechage we were allowed to catch up with the 60-strong Australian contingent that had travelled to Beijing to support us. During the Games, the rules regarding access to the outside world are quite clear. You are not allowed to leave the village or have anyone visit you without authorisation, and at the venues you need to stay within the designated athletes' area. But for fifteen minutes we were allowed to hug and kiss and talk to the people we cared most about, and it was a better tonic than anything else the Chinese officials could have arranged.

During the heat and the repechage we could see our support base sitting in the stands on the side of the course wearing bright yellow T-shirts with the names Kat and John emblazoned on them. We could hear them cheering, and screaming out chants like 'Aussie, Aussie, Aussie, oi, oi, oi!' There were members of my family, Kathryn's family, our friends and other supporters, including about a hundred people from China I'd never met in my life, who were wearing their own John Maclean T-shirts and carrying John Maclean flags. They worked for the Beijing office of Datacraft, who are owned by Dimension Data, the company I consult for in Sydney.

Among the crowd were my two best friends, Johnno and David Knight. My mentor and friend Marc Robinson had flown in especially for the event from the United States, with his wife Lori. There was my brother Marc, who'd come all the way from New Zealand, and my half-brother Don, from Canada. And then there was Amanda, my love, my fiancée and my future, the woman I wish to spend the rest of my life with and create a family. People often asked me what my next event would be after this, and I'd tell them, 'I'm settling down. I want a gold-medal marriage.' It was important that Amanda be here to see this, the capping of my professional sporting career, and when we won the final she would be the first person I would want to see.

Many of the people who have come to Beijing have been with me from the start of my professional sporting career until now, the end of it. Having them here is a great way to finish. I believe that I'm doing it for all of them, who have given of themselves to support me in so many different ways over the years. It's my way of saying, 'Thank you for helping me to dream and live the life I wanted.'

A great man I know believes that the patients who move on successfully with their lives after spinal cord injuries are the ones who are prepared to share their journey with others. His name is John Yeo, and he ran the spinal unit at the Royal North Shore Hospital in Sydney for nearly thirty years. He was in charge when I was admitted in 1988 and we still keep in touch. I can't remember the day when I took his advice about sharing the journey to heart, but he's right, of course. I have drawn strength from positive people, and I have had my greatest successes after building a team of like-minded souls around me.

The moment of truth has arrived: 11 September 2008. I can see from the morning sky that it's going to be a hot, sunny day. At the village I'm trying to stay as relaxed as possible. But I'm nervous. After eighteen months of living and breathing this event, it now comes down to less than five minutes of racing. This is it.

Pedro came to see Kathryn and me early that morning. He thought we should change our race plan. He believed we needed to go out with a higher stroke rate, higher than we'd ever done before, to try to keep up with China. It was a risky strategy. Without training for it, we couldn't be sure we wouldn't fall apart at the back end of the race. Kat and I discussed the change and decided that, after eighteen months of training to a particular plan, to make such a change now left us vulnerable. We decided to stick with what we knew. We would go out at 42, bring it down to 36, stay strong and mow them down at the back end. We planned to pick up Brazil between the 500 and 750 metres, and our race with China would start at the 750 mark.

If we stick to our race plan I know we will beat China and it will happen just before we cross the finish line.

Last-minute chats about changing an established race plan are unsettling. For rowers who have grown up in boats and raced with different plans on different occasions, it might be okay. But we didn't have that bank of experience. I knew Kathryn was trying to be relaxed but that China's convincing win in the heat was playing on her mind. I tried to reassure her. 'Kathryn, if we stick to this plan, we will win. You've got to get a sense of this. We will win.'

We left for the venue around 2 pm. Our bus had a police escort front and back. Kathryn sat next to me but we didn't talk much. I didn't want to invade her space, and I don't think she wanted to invade mine. Richard Bennett, the Australian team's sports psychologist, sat behind us. We'd had an hour's session with him on the second day. He was a surfer and a very cool guy. He just said, 'Be relaxed and confident within yourselves. Make sure you get the blade in where you need to get it in and just let it run. Do what you guys do.'

When we arrived at the course, we made our way through the check-in area and headed down to the boat shed. We had some time to kill and I spent mine reading a book called *The Adversity Advantage*, by Erik Weihenmayer and Paul Stoltz. Weihenmayer is the only blind man in history to reach the seven summits, the tallest peak on every continent, including Everest. Stolz has spent years decoding the human relationship with adversity, and their book draws business analogies around how people can use adversity as a positive force. I like books with inspirational messages and quotes and I thought it was a good thing to have on hand.

When the time comes, I go to the change-room, pull on my zootie and put some Vaseline under my arms. Pedro says to us, 'Concentrate on your technique and make sure you pull hard through the stroke. Be sharp front and back.' Then he says, 'Someone is going to have to say something at a crucial time. The crucial word is "now", and Kathryn will say it at the 500.' We head down to the pontoon and the boat. It's now about twenty minutes to race time and I can see the flash of yellow shirts in the stands. Our supporters are making so much noise that everyone can hear their chants and whistling. I remember Drew Ginn telling me that when my body started hurting at the 750 metre mark to use the crowd to get me over the line. I now understand what he means.

We start rowing towards the warm-up area. I see the Australian flags draped over the stand and think, 'Okay, this is pretty special, this is what we've been training for.' I worked out a long time ago with Kathryn not to talk to her in the boat. If there is any communication at all, it is perfunctory. We do a 20-stroke piece and then a 10-stroke piece and a few practice starts, making sure we are up at the bridge with about fifteen minutes to go.

We are away. At the 250-metre mark Brazil is in front. We are clear in second place, with China breathing down our necks in third. At 500 metres, Brazil is still in front, but now China is in second place. Kathryn says, 'Now!' Italy, Great Britain and Poland are out of contention. At the 750 mark, China hits the front. We are in second place and Brazil has slipped back to third. It's a two-boat race. Can we make up the difference?

Australia, China, Australia, China. Next thing I know is the beep that signals the finish line.

I look over to lane 3 and know instinctively we didn't make it. Despite our greatest efforts, we have come second—but only by the smallest of margins. After 1000 metres, only 0.89 seconds, no more than two metres, separated us.

I slap Kathryn's hand in a sort of high five and slump forward, sucking oxygen into my lungs. We've given it everything. That's what I call 100 per cent—but I am devastated. Kathryn has her hand in the air acknowledging the crowd and our silver-medal performance, but I feel as though something I really want has been within my reach, only to be taken away just as I grasp for it.

Everyone who knew me knew how much I was hurting. My focus was always winning the gold medal and when it didn't happen, the pain of disappointment was worse than the pain in my aching arms. In the grandstand, among my family and friends, the mood was one of stunned realisation. Johnno went downstairs to cry, he felt so bad for me. It takes a lot to bring him to tears. He knew the reason I was here—everyone knew the reason I was here. I wanted the fairytale ending; I wanted to go out with a gold medal. But as I have learnt so acutely in my life, it is what it is, and you can't turn back the clock.

I've always said to kids in wheelchairs, 'Look what you can do. You can dream, believe and achieve. You can be as competitive as anyone else in your classroom, your suburb, your country and the world.' I had wanted to say that the next time with a gold medal to share.

People had asked me what would happen if I didn't win. Would life go on if I didn't win gold? 'Absolutely,' I'd say. 'If there's no gold medal, there's no gold medal. Whatever happens,

I will have come a long way from where I first started out in this sport. I've been around the block a few times. I know what it's like to get hit by a truck and to crash at the Olympic Games, so I know what disappointment is all about and not getting what you want. But it's about putting yourself in the game. It's about putting your foot in the water and having a go.'

CHAPTER FIFTEEN

A SENSE OF CLOSURE

'I have seen many motivational speakers and they are usually very extroverted people with the "Ra Ra" attitude to fire-up the troops. The difference with John is he touches people with his story in a very modest and humble way. He has clearly earned the right to be up there'
—MARC ROBINSON, FRIEND AND MENTOR

I didn't return to the athletes' village. I had already packed my bags before the rowing final and that night I checked into the hotel where Amanda and most of my friends and family were staying. Amanda and I spent the next few days with them in Beijing before heading to Shanghai, where I got measured for the suit I planned to wear at our wedding. I also bought a wedding band that, coincidentally, had been made in Beijing, and could joke that 'Yes, I did pick up gold in Beijing'.

Everyone knew the truth—I was bitterly disappointed about the outcome of the race. I had already announced my retirement from competitive sport and it was no secret I wanted to end my professional career with gold. Some of my friends quietly raised the possibility of going to the London Paralympics in 2012, but I couldn't see it happening. The fire in my belly had finally gone out.

When I returned to Australia a week later I was facing a different future. One that included marriage to the woman I loved, hopefully some children on the not-too-distant horizon, and growing my own business doing what I'm good at—talking to people and helping them realise their full potential. I was moving from one world to another, and while it was exciting and I looked forward to it immensely I still had some unfinished business with my past. The last thing I wanted to do was embark on a new chapter in my life when I hadn't quite finished writing the last one.

I wanted to find the truck driver whose vehicle hit me all those years ago. I had no idea how such a meeting would pan out. I didn't know what he'd say, or how he'd react to me or how I'd feel when I met him in person, face-to-face for the first time. I would be lying if I didn't say the uncertainty of it unsettled me. It did.

I also knew that if I didn't face up to this I would never be free of it.

I became an incomplete paraplegic because of a road accident. Running was the thing I loved to do most in life and it was taken away from me in a split second without warning or consultation. I would give away everything I have—the success I've enjoyed as an athlete, the international travel and sporting experiences and the money I've earned—and go live in a tin shed and eat potatoes for the rest of my life if I could only have the use of my legs again. I would swap it right now. I'd say, 'Yes, let's go, I'm ready to do it.' I'd probably do what Forrest Gump did in the movie, I'd run and run and run because I have twenty years worth of running to catch up on. I know Amanda wouldn't love me any less if I had nothing to my name and was mowing lawns for a living.

I don't often talk about the pain I am constantly in, but it's one of the legacies of the horrific injuries I suffered that day. My bony bum gets really sore if I sit too long and my right foot suffers hypersensitivity, and now there's some arthritis in the ankle. That means they ache, dreadfully some nights, so when I'm in bed I curl up into the foetal position with a pillow between my legs, holding my foot. I've done this since the accident. I don't know why, but it seems to give some respite from the pain.

With intense exercise, the pain in my left shoulder also increases. I suspect I triggered an injury doing the first Ironman in '95, and the pain and stiffness has got progressively worse as the years have gone by. I depend on my arms like a kidney patient is reliant on dialysis and can't imagine my life or how I would cope with it if anything were to happen to them. Having investigated an operation and been advised against it, at the moment I put up with the pain and discomfort.

Most people work to earn money so they can enjoy a certain lifestyle. Maybe that's a nice house, new car, good holidays and the flexibility to eat out at a restaurant occasionally. Because of the pain I am in a lot of the time, for me it's all about comfort. Money represents relief from pain—a better seat on a plane, a decent hotel with a firm mattress, a hatchback car for my wheelchair and a deep bath at home with easy access.

Meeting the man who put me in a wheelchair was not going to be easy. I didn't feel anger towards him or crave retribution, but I was apprehensive about getting in touch with him, hearing his voice, seeing him in person. My concern was that it might be a negative experience—and that would make things worse for me, not better. I understand why people bury incidents from their past deep in the recesses of their mind, locked down and almost impenetrable. But I also knew that if I didn't face up to this I would never be free of it. I wanted to know what happened in the cabin of that truck just before it hit me and what the driver's reaction had been and how his own life had turned out. I wanted to know for sure that it was an accident, that my paraplegia was an unfortunate consequence of a random event. Accidents happen in life all the time—I accept that—but I needed to hear him say that's what it was.

I couldn't help but think of what Maurie Rayner would have said about taking this step now, so long after it all happened. 'Now, that's a big yuck bit of your life!'—I could almost hear him saying it. He would have endorsed a meeting, I'm sure. He was right when he said those 'yuck bits' weigh us down and prevent us moving forward with our lives. If I could meet the truck driver and find out just what happened that day, if I could face up to him and whatever explanation he might give me, if I could find it in my heart to forgive him, then it would be worthwhile. I wouldn't have to lock him away in a no-go zone in the back of my mind and that would help me finish this chapter of my life.

It is one thing deciding you want to meet someone after twenty years and another thing altogether finding that person. I didn't know if the truck driver even wanted to be found. Maybe he dreaded the day when he picked up the phone and I was on the other end, so he had taken steps to prevent that from ever happening. I am not skilled at this sort of work so I turned to Lynne Cossar. Lynne and I have spent many hours going through my life in painstaking detail to put this book together. She understood exactly what this meeting meant to me. I was confronting my greatest fear and she was mindful of that. 'Can you find him?' I asked her. 'I think it's possible to find anyone,' she said. 'It will depend on whether he wants to be found. Are you sure this is what you want to do?' This seemed like an odd question, given the long conversations we'd had about the accident and how I felt about it, but the moment I said 'Yes I'm sure', I knew exactly why she had asked. Once the words were spoken out loud there was no turning back. Wheels had been put in motion. It was like I had boarded a train and there was no stopping until I reached my destination.

The search for the truck driver (let's just call him Tom, which of course is not his name) began in earnest by turning to the largest contact book in the world, the phone book, or, more accurately in this case, White Pages Online. Was it possible we would get lucky and his name would be there, clearly and simply, and I could just pick up the phone and it would be done? Could it be that easy? No. There were people listed with the same family name, but no one with the same initials. I didn't want to be cold-calling people who might even turn out to be his children. I wanted more control over the process, more certainty over who I was speaking to when they answered their phone.

'Let's narrow the search then,' Lynne said. Armed with Tom's full name, and his address at the time of the accident, which we knew from the Supreme Court case file I'd accessed earlier, Lynne went to the State Library of NSW to search the electoral roll on microfiche. Voting is compulsory in Australia and most people aged eighteen or older are registered because you are fined if you don't register.

I couldn't help but think how many secrets must be housed in that building. Alphabetised in phone books and filing cabinets were the names, addresses and phone numbers of millions of Australians, dating back decades. Could you hide, even if you wanted to? Lynne had told me that it could take a few days to search the material. When she finally called me after office hours on the third afternoon, I felt on edge. 'Tom's not on the current electoral roll, John,' Lynne said. I felt disappointed. Having made the decision to contact him, the prospect of not being able to find him left me feeling despondent. 'What now, then?' I asked. Lynne explained that she had gone back to the date of the accident and tracked him from there. He had lived in the same house until 1993, moved, moved again in late 1994 or early 1995. He dropped off the radar completely in 1999. 'There's more,' she said. 'John, the house he lived in when he was last registered to vote is only one suburb away from you. He was living that close for more than three years and it's only a few kilometres from the scene of the accident—which he must have driven past almost every day.' I had long since made my peace with the guardrail on the M4—which according to one eyewitness I landed on after being catapulted through the air—and drove past it myself most days of the week. That didn't trouble me. The fact that Tom had lived only a suburb away did. Had I seen him at Penrith Plaza and not known who he was? Did he know me? I had attracted a good deal of publicity after the Hawaii Ironman and my Channel crossing, especially in the local paper, which he most likely would have seen. How did he feel about that? Was there any significance to his moving there?

Suddenly, more questions were raised than answered. I was amazed at the picture those records had painted and what they told me about his life. I found it odd that he had been on the electoral roll for more than ten years and then dropped off it. Was he dead? Could that be possible? Or had he moved overseas? Then came more news: 'John! I think I've found his parents—and I have their phone number.'

They were listed on the electoral roll, with the same family name, at the same address as Tom at the time of the accident. They had moved several times since then and still lived together, albeit in a different state. 'It has to be his mum and dad,' Lynne said. 'I'm sure of it.' I said nothing for a while as I digested this information and weighed up what I felt about it. 'I'll call them,' I said.

I had not anticipated a third party being involved and was aware that his parents must be getting on in years. I didn't want to cause them undue distress by dragging unpleasant parts of the past out of the closet, but it was the best lead we had and I was now determined to follow this through. Tom was becoming more real to me by the minute, and I started framing the questions I would put to his mum or dad, depending on who answered the phone.

I would be lying if I said I dialled the number effortlessly. I was nervous and I'm sure my voice faltered slightly when an older man answered the phone after only a couple of rings. 'Hello,' he said. 'Hello,' I replied. 'My name's John Maclean. I wanted to touch base with you. Many years ago I was involved in an accident. I was riding my pushbike on the M4 when I got hit by a truck. There is no malice in this call, but I believe your son may have been the driver of the truck. It's twenty years since the accident and I just wanted to meet with your son. There are no hard feelings from my side. I just want to connect with him if I can. I hope you don't mind me ringing up out of the blue?'

The phone line was deafeningly quiet for a few seconds, before the voice on the other end said, 'It's a bit of a shock.' No denial or fobbing me off. It was the truck driver's father for sure. 'I'm sorry about that,' I said. 'Things have moved on for me and I just wanted to make sure they were okay with your son and to see how things unfolded for him.' 'You're looking for where he's living?' The father sounded like he was in his seventies, and he was as sharp as a tack. He had cut to the chase immediately and I admired him for that. 'Yeah,' I said. 'I wanted to see whether he might be interested in meeting face to face.' 'I'm afraid I can't answer that for you,' the father said. 'Obviously he doesn't live with us these days and it's a long while ago now and I'm just not sure how he is. Before I can give anything to you I'd have to talk to him, I'm pretty sure.'

No father would volunteer his son's phone number to someone with a story like mine without checking first. I appreciated that, and I'd expected it. 'Yeah, that's a good idea,' I replied. 'Is he living in Australia or is he overseas?' 'No, he's still in Australia, but he gets around a bit. We don't see him all that often. If you want to give me a number, next time I'm in contact with him I'll put it to him and give him your number.' I recited my mobile number and asked one final question: 'When do you think you might speak with him?' 'Probably some time this weekend.' 'Thanks for taking the call,' I said, and before I got the words out the father had hung up.

It was done but I felt no sense of satisfaction. I had established that Tom was alive and living in Australia, but I had effectively surrendered control of my search to him. Once his dad gave him my number, he was in the driver's seat. He could ring me whenever he wanted, day or night, in a week's time, in a month or in a year, and every time my mobile signalled an incoming call I'd be looking at the number to see if I recognised it and wondering whether it was Tom on the other end. Worse still, he could choose not to call, and I wasn't sure I could deal with that. It had taken so much soul-searching and courage to finally decide to meet him that to never get the opportunity was something I didn't want to contemplate.

I lost control of my life for a long time after the accident. I lost control of my legs forever. While I don't sweat the small things anymore, and I never look to control the things I can't, I do like to be organised and planned. The fact that the person who had affected my life more than anyone else now had control of when contact between us would be made was unsettling for me. Crazy as it might sound, I couldn't help thinking that the balance between us had shifted and that threw out my equilibrium.

It was a waiting game. 'The ball's in Tom's court now,' I told Lynne. 'Not necessarily, John,' she replied. 'There's always another way.' She explained that while I waited for his call she would exhaust the other lead we had, the addresses when he was still listed on the electoral roll. 'I'll doorknock the streets and see if anyone remembers him. You never know.' And that's what she did—three separate streets in different parts of Sydney. We were like detectives tracking down leads and trying to think as laterally as we could about where we could look next. Lynne's doorknocking produced nothing except sore knuckles and a few uncomfortable encounters with aggressive dogs. 'It's been too long,' she told me. The trail had gone cold.

Two weeks went by and there was still no call. It was almost certain that Tom's father had told him about me by now. I had to assume Tom had my phone number and was either still thinking about calling me or had decided against it. I hadn't really expected his father would get in touch with me but privately I was hoping that if he'd had the conversation with his son and the response was, 'No way! I don't want anything to do with it,' then he might find it in his heart to let me know. Surely he understood how much I was sweating on the phone call? I was grasping at straws, and I knew it.

'Do you think he could be in gaol?' Lynne said to me, and promptly started calling all the state Correctional Services Departments. I was surprised they gave out that sort of information but they do and, no, Tom wasn't incarcerated.

I was losing all hope when I remembered I had a friend in the police force. I rang him on the off-chance he might be able to recommend another line of inquiry. 'I can't look him up on our data base,' he told me. 'It's against our rules and they audit all our calls. Have you applied for the accident report?' 'I have,' I said. 'When that comes through look for other leads, like the company he worked for and old colleagues and work mates. I'm sorry there's nothing else I can do for you, but keep in touch.' 'Thanks mate,' I replied. The fact was I had already been sent the accident report after applying for it through Freedom of Information. It provided nothing new and while I had requested all statements, witness interviews and photos, I'd received none of that. When I rang the FoI unit to find out why, I was told I'd been given everything they had, and that there was no point lodging an appeal.

I tried a couple of times to ring Tom's father back, but when the calls went through to voicemail I decided against leaving messages. I was concerned about getting him involved, mainly because of his age. I was starting to think that meeting Tom just wasn't meant to be when Lynne called with news: 'John, I've found him on Facebook!'

Logging on myself as we spoke, I came face to face with a childhood snap of a person with the same family name and first name. 'How can you be sure it's him?' I asked. 'It's just a feeling. It's the same name and it's not a common one. And look at his friends. Most of them are around your age.' I had a vague memory that the truck driver was a couple of years younger than me. I think the policeman who'd attended the accident and kept in touch with me over the years told me that, and I had shared the information with Lynne. Still, the age of the friends on his Facebook page seemed a tenuous link, but it was the only other lead we had. I thought, 'Should I email him?' By now he knew I was looking for him, so how would that help? 'We need to narrow the search again,' Lynne said. And with that she went back to the State Library, and to the electoral roll, with the list of names from the site.

No addresses are ever listed on Facebook, just names and country of origin. But using the electoral roll Lynne matched names with addresses, cross-referenced them with names on White Pages Online, and started ringing around Australia. A couple of days and more than a hundred phone calls later she rang me: 'John, I have his phone numbers—work and mobile.' 'Are you sure?' I said. 'I'm positive,' she replied. 'I got the work number off a friend of his and then rang the company and they gave me his mobile number. It's him, John. There's no doubt.' I wrote the numbers down and stared at them for a long, long time. I found it a spine-chilling prospect that I could pick up the phone and within seconds be hearing Tom's voice on the other end.

At no stage did Lynne divulge the reason for her calls. We were always mindful of Tom's privacy, and saw no benefit in putting him offside from the start. I had no idea how many people he had told about the accident, but you would have to assume it was not something he broadcast about himself. It was not my intention to make his life more difficult.

Dialling that number was extremely difficult. It was nothing compared to facing up to the injuries I'd suffered when I woke up in the spinal unit at Royal North Shore Hospital, but I had no choice but to keep going then. It was different to competing in the Hawaii Ironman and swimming the English Channel. They were challenges over which I had some control. It was different to crashing at the 2000 Olympic Games and coming second at the 2008 Beijing Paralympic Games when all I wanted was gold. They were sporting events and I learnt a long time ago that life goes on after such experiences. Facing the man who put me in a wheelchair was another issue altogether. I couldn't control what was going to happen next—what he would say, whether he would agree to a meeting. I would be putting the ball squarely in his court and that was both risky and confronting.

As I picked up my Blackberry and punched in the digits of the mobile number my hand was trembling and my mouth was dry. I was accustomed to nerves before big sporting events, but the feeling that was sweeping over me was more gut-wrenching than anything I'd ever encountered. The phone rang, and rang and rang, and then I heard Tom's voice for the first time. 'Leave a message,' he said. I didn't, of course. I broke the connection and sat looking at my Blackberry for what seemed like an age. I tried to imagine the face that belonged to that voice, whether he'd check for missed calls and discover I'd been ringing him. Had he added my number to his address book so when I rang my name flashed on screen? Or was he just not available to take the call?

I didn't feel up to ringing again straight away. I wanted to feel more composed so I left it for the day and rang the next morning. The mobile went straight through to voicemail, so I tried the work number. Tom wasn't available so I left a message with the receptionist. I now felt I had a lot at stake. I wanted to meet him. I wanted for everything between us to be aired and finally put to rest. I had come this far, and there was no turning back. I tried his mobile again. It rang a couple of times before he picked up. 'Hello,' he said. 'Hello, my name is John Maclean,' I replied. 'I have been trying to get in touch with you for a while. I rang your dad recently. I am at a stage of my life where I am moving forward and I was hoping we could meet. I have no intention of malice but it would help me with closure.'

There, I had said it—blurted it out, more precisely—before he had the chance to hang up. My heart was beating so fast and loud I could hear it thumping through my shirt. 'I am okay with that,' Tom said. No objection or questions, just five words in a non-committal tone. The phone was no place for this conversation so we arranged to meet the following week. I would fly to the city he was living in and we'd meet at a hotel I knew. I was keen to get it over with now, and I didn't want to give him a chance to change his mind.

Oddly enough, I think I felt more nervous before making the call than I did before meeting him. I didn't tell many people what I was doing, just said I had some business interstate. Amanda knew, of course, and David Knight and Johnno. David rang me when I was in the Qantas Club lounge at Sydney Airport just to check I was okay with everything. Hearing his voice made me smile. I reminded myself again how lucky I was to have such good people in my life.

The flight was uneventful. I hired a car when I arrived and checked the map so I knew where I was going. I had booked a suite at the hotel. We were to rendezvous in the lobby at midday, but I thought it would be good to have a separate space to go to, not to mention some privacy. The sun was shining and it was a beautiful, clear morning but I barely noticed as I negotiated my way out of the airport and into the heavy mid-morning traffic.

I wanted to get there and get it over with. I reached the hotel an hour early and picked up the keys to the room before heading to the restaurant to have an orange juice and watch the minutes tick by. A million thoughts were racing through my head, but I tried to clear my mind and concentrate on what I wanted out of this exercise—some clarity around what happened and some answers. About 11.45 I wheeled into the lobby and transferred into a lounge chair facing the entrance. I wanted to see Tom walk in and the look on his face when he saw me for the first time. I knew he would recognise me—the wheelchair parked beside me would make sure of that. But I had a gut feeling I would know him too. I wondered what he was thinking—and for one brief moment I thought, 'I wonder if he will turn up at all.'

I saw him coming even before he had reached the automatic glass entrance doors. I had no idea what he looked like but something told me it was definitely him. Maybe it was the purposeful way he walked into the hotel, although there was a distinct air of nervousness in his movements. Maybe it was the almost furtive way he scanned the room, or the flushed, red glow enveloping his face. It only took a few seconds before his gaze fixed on me and he started towards me. I transferred into my wheelchair so that I could move towards him, almost like I was meeting him halfway. 'Hello Tom, I'm John,' I said. 'Thanks for coming.' He extended his hand and we shook.

I had rehearsed what I would say in an attempt to put him at ease. The first few seconds of any meeting are critical and I wanted to take the edge off any discomfort he might be feeling. I wanted answers and his cooperation, and I was not going to get that by being surly. This was not about retribution or anger. It was about closure and forgiveness. I wanted both of us to leave the hotel feeling our meeting had been a positive experience. I wanted to make it work.

He looked really nervous and jittery, and suddenly I realised how much courage it had taken for him to come here today. I wondered if he'd thought about turning around and leaving on the spot, but he hadn't done it and I appreciated that. I told him I had arranged a suite where we could talk in private, and steered him towards the lift and the third floor. We made polite small talk on the way. I asked whether he'd taken the day off, and he said, 'How was your flight?' We both wanted to avoid an awkward silence before our real conversation began. He didn't baulk at getting into the lift. I think he felt relieved that no one would be able to overhear our coming discussion.

Unlocking the door to the room, I invited Tom to sit where he felt most comfortable. He took up a position on the three-seater lounge with his back to the window. I transferred into a lounge chair facing him. He crossed his legs and kept his hands clenched in his lap as he waited for me to start. I had been correct about his age. He was younger than me, but I got the impression his life had not been easy. Wearing dark pants and a striped business shirt unbuttoned at the neck, he looked as though he'd weathered more than his fair share of ups and downs.

I thanked him again for coming and explained that I had been revisiting parts of my life in an attempt to get closure. 'The last part of the jigsaw was to finally meet you and get your interpretation of how things unfolded. What was your recollection of the accident?'

Tom drew a deep breath and shifted a little on the lounge. I felt he was choosing his words carefully. From the moment he started talking I got the distinct impression he had rehearsed the answer, anticipating what the first question would be. 'I was driving down the highway and was coming up on the back of another truck and I was signalling and wanting to go out and around,' he said rather nervously. 'I don't remember hearing anything. And I don't remember seeing a cyclist, I was looking in my side-view mirror and didn't realise anything had happened until I saw this guy on the motorbike coming up beside me waving at me with one hand and motioning for me to pull over. I first knew something had happened was when I got out and walked around and saw the front of the truck. From my recollection [the force of impact] bent the bullbar and half dented the front of the truck. The guy on the motorbike was the first person that spoke to me and then a car pulled up behind as well.'

I knew most of this from the accident report. I asked Tom if he'd seen me on the side of the road or walked back to where I was lying. I had a photograph of the scene that showed four people looking shell-shocked as ambulance officers worked on me. I had wondered if Tom was one of those people, but he said, 'No. I didn't walk back. I stayed where the truck was. I believe someone told me to stay up there, not to go back because there were enough people already doing what they could. I stayed with the truck until the police came. I was shaking, I think, and sitting on the guardrail.'

His words corroborated what the policeman who attended the accident had told me, that when he'd approached the truck driver he was sitting by the side of the freeway with his head cradled in his hands. 'I can recall he was very upset,' the policeman said. 'And I suppose a little defensive of himself at the time, not knowing what the consequences of his actions would be. He was concerned for you, John.'

I was thinking about this when Tom's voice jolted me back to the moment. He said he stayed with the truck until the police approached him. 'From what I remember of the process we were probably there on the side of the road for a couple of hours,' he said. 'I went back to the police station with them [the police] and was probably there for another couple of hours. I don't remember whether they charged me straight away or not. I remember going to the police station, giving the police statement and I remember them taking me back to the truck and I continued on and finished my delivery. I drove out to Penrith, unloaded and drove back to Parramatta. I parked the truck and sat there and waited till someone else turned up, and fell apart, basically. I was driven home from work. They wouldn't let me drive.'

There were a few moments of silence as I thought about what he'd said. It struck me as odd that they wouldn't let him drive home from the depot, but hours before that he had climbed back into the same truck that had broken so many bones in my body and finished his run. He was delivering empty fire extinguishers, but usually he shifted furniture, he said. Maybe he kept his composure until he arrived somewhere he felt safe. Maybe there is something to the accepted wisdom that when you fall off a horse you should jump back on it straight away or you lose your nerve to ever do so. Was that why the police had driven him back to the truck? These thoughts were swirling through my mind when Tom interrupted and told me again how upset he'd been at the depot. He'd fallen apart and was crying, he said. His voice had dropped and there was quietness about his tone that took me a little by surprise. When he first started talking about the accident it was as if he were in a court room, but now Tom was looking at me directly, eye to eye, and I knew it wasn't easy for him recalling that scene at the depot. 'I actually remember that we rang the hospital to see what was happening with you,' he said. 'They obviously wouldn't tell us anything but I do remember my supervisor making the call. I was driven home after that and then I had a few days off.'

I knew immediately what was to follow—the question that I always wanted answered. 'What about the hospital?' I said as evenly as I could. 'Was there a thought of going to the hospital?' 'There was certainly a thought,' he said, a little nervously, as if he understood this was an issue for me. 'When the boss actually found out what had happened he told me to stay away. So I just left it at that. The subject was not discussed again within the working environment.'

So he was warned off any contact. 'Do you think [the boss] did that for legal reasons or because he just wanted you to get on with it and forget about it?' I pressed. This was important to me. I had lain in RNS for many weeks, expecting the truck driver to walk through the door at any moment. I had waited for him, listened for his footsteps even. Tom paused slightly, cleared his throat and said, 'Personally, I think it was a bit of both. I think it may well have been to some extent more legal reasons. But you know, I believe it was also partly to try to get over it.'

When I'd first decided to make contact with Tom I'd made a mental list of the things I wanted to achieve from meeting him. It wasn't a long list. I had thought if he explained it was an accident and he was sorry for what had happened, that would suffice. What more could I reasonably expect? What more did I need? I was wrong. I now understood that *I* needed to say something to *him*. *I* needed to get something off *my* chest. I took a deep breath and started down a path I never thought I'd be travelling.

'Thank you for giving me your thoughts,' I said. 'Part of me—a big part of me—was waiting for you to come in and say, "I'm sorry." Accidents happen every day and that would have been good for me to hear at that time. People have said to me, "What happened with the truck driver?" and I'd say, "I don't know, I never met him." I know drivers don't like pushbikes on the freeway. I couldn't process what happened because I didn't know and I ended up speculating. I suppose if the shoe were on the other foot—that's often how I think—if the roles were reversed and I was advised not to go [to the hospital] I would have disregarded that advice and still gone in for my own peace of mind. Even if people weren't happy for that to take place, I would have gone, "Hey, that's something that I need to do." I would like to have had access to you at that time. It would have been good for me to face you.'

There, I had said it. After twenty years the words were finally out in the open. I looked at Tom and for a brief moment I saw his eyes mist over. He was on the verge of tears and for the first time I realised that he had not escaped the incident unscathed either even though he had moved so quickly to try to put it behind him. His voice faltered briefly before he continued: 'Why did it happen?' he asked, as if he were searching for a reason for it. 'What caused it? What could I have done to not make it happen? I don't know. I don't believe there is an answer to that. I don't believe anyone can give you an answer to that. I don't dwell on it. Maybe I have tried to block it out. Again, maybe that comes back to the fact that it is something I don't feel proud of that's happened in my life.'

Neither of us said anything for a few moments. Tom's head had dropped and he was looking at his hands. I was the one that broke the silence. I asked how old he was at the time. 'I was twenty or something like that,' he replied, leaning back in the lounge. 'I would have been driving for twelve months at that stage. It's hard to get someone who's under twenty-five driving a truck now, purely for insurance reasons, you know. Obviously it's an expensive exercise. So yeah, I was certainly young to drive a truck. Did I work hard? At times I'm sure I did. For me, I guess I was a truck driver because I didn't know what else to be, quite frankly. I drove for another eight years. Actually I became a driving instructor, partly because that was the next step in the career but also to try to improve what I saw on the road. I spent a lot of time in trucks. I've heard a lot of stories about truck drivers driving between Sydney and Brisbane in eight hours and I've thought about the speeds they must be doing to achieve that time frame. You can't do that these days. In some ways I was probably looking to have some effect on what people do—I thought that would be a good thing.'

The times I had thought of the truck driver I wondered how the accident had affected him and his family. Did it prevent him from moving forward with his life? Did it haunt him in his dreams? It was not something that I imagined he could easily forget, and its impact on him was something I was keen to know. 'What effect did it have on you?' I asked, half expecting to hear how it had altered the course of his life. I wasn't at all prepared for the answer. 'To be quite honest, I don't know if there was any great effect at all,' he replied quickly. I looked at his face and knew he was telling the truth. He did not flinch and his gaze was direct. 'I was quite involved in the church back then. I had a good support group around me, I guess. I remember consulting a lawyer and going to court. The lawyer said "plead guilty", and I didn't understand much. I don't remember the court case really. I was charged with negligent driving and I think I was fined. I don't really remember. I didn't lose my licence.'

It struck me then that maybe Tom had been able to block out the accident so completely because he had never seen me lying lifeless on the road or bruised and battered in the hospital bed. If he had been able to put a face to the name or in this case an image to the accident maybe it would have made a difference. I would never know. I also found his recollection— or lack thereof—of the court case odd, but thought it might be a no-go area for him. It occurred to me there might be certain details he didn't wish to share, and that was okay.

Tom told me he had no idea whether I had lived or died until later on when he went to court. 'I don't know if it was necessarily the police that told me,' he said, pausing briefly and rubbing his chin with his fingers as if he was trying to prompt a memory. 'I think it may well have been the time I was going to court. I don't remember anyone giving us any updates of what happened, what hospital you were in. It was probably some time around 1991 that I found out you were alive.' 'Didn't you ever wonder?' I asked, a little incredulous that anyone would not want to know what had happened. If it were me I would have had to find out or it would have been on my mind constantly. 'Oh, look, I'm sure I did, but it's not something I remember sitting and thinking about. It must have been 1991 or 1992, I think, when I found out for sure.'

I didn't see the point in pressing Tom on this, mainly because his memory seemed so sketchy, but it crossed my mind he probably knew I survived when he went to court on the negligent driving charge. If I had died the charge may well have been different. He certainly would have been aware of my injuries—my paraplegia—after my lawyers filed suit for compensation. Our paths never crossed in court, but he would have been required to give evidence.

What you hold onto in life holds onto you.

Tom said it was a few years after that he saw me on television and put two and two together. 'I remember you talking about the accident on a freeway and a truck and where it was and that's when the name connected with me and I thought, "Hang on, I know that story, I was the driver of that truck." I don't remember what year that was but that's certainly what happened. Realising who you were at the time made me think that it was me who did that. I guess that shocked me.' Tom paused before continuing: 'It was good to see that you were out there achieving some goals. They're things I would never be able to achieve.'

I asked if he'd ever considered getting in touch with me. 'Has that ever crossed your mind?' Tom seemed to relax a little now that the conversation had moved away from the accident and the legal aftermath. 'It's probably come up a couple of times in the last six to eight years when I saw you on television,' he said. 'But at the same time I guess I didn't know whether it was my place to do that. I was the one driving the truck. I'm not the one that's been affected by it greatly. If I knew it was going to happen, I would have avoided it. It's certainly not something that I set out to do. I didn't know if you wanted to go back. I didn't know if I had the right to bring it up. When my father rang me and told me you had called he said, "I don't know if you want to do this." I guess it was at that point I thought, "Yes, I want to do it." I wanted to go and say "Sorry", that if I could do anything different I would.'

And there it was! He had finally used the word 'sorry'. Tom hadn't looked me in the eye and said it directly to my face. But he had said it, even if in a roundabout way, and I believed he was. We had been talking for more than an hour and I knew it was not going to turn into an Oprah Winfrey-type couch experience, where he burst into tears and we hugged and he said 'sorry' over and over again and lamented how it had completely ruined his life. All that had transpired between us in terms of the impact we'd had on each other's lives was not going to be erased after one meeting. But the sting had gone out of it, at least for me.

At that moment I was struck by how real this experience was. It was neither disappointing nor completely gratifying. It was what it was, and suddenly that seemed okay to me. Tom had his pride, and I believe he went as far as he could go. We are men. And while close female friends have since asked about that conversation and expressed amazement at what they claim is unresolved pain, I liked the fact that we talked and went as far with each other as we could. I didn't want to become his friend, nor he mine, I suspect. I wasn't his counsellor. We had briefly danced with each other around an event in our lives that was as sensitive as I could imagine any life experience could be, notwithstanding the death of a child. Looking at Tom now, I respected the magnitude of what we had achieved today. It was, as I'd hoped, a cathartic experience for me.

I couldn't help then but ask about his family. 'Did your parents ever revisit the accident?' I said. 'I don't remember it ever having been a topic of discussion,' he replied, looking down at his hands. 'I know that my father was a little bit apprehensive about bringing it up. I guess in some respects, yes, the family is close but I come from an English family and we don't show much love. Everyone knows that we are a family and we all get on, but you know, I don't think he quite knew how to handle it at the time. I can't say that I told him I was meeting you but I certainly will when next we speak in our weekly phone call. I will let him know that I have got together with you.'

Tom told me he'd been surprised I'd finally contacted him. 'It has been a long time,' he said. 'When you asked if I wanted to meet I was like "Yeah, I think I want to do that." I've been through different things in my life, different to yours, and I guess I reflect and appreciate the way people are these days and I think I needed to come and find out what your life has really been like. I think about [the accident]. Not every day, but certainly when your name is mentioned on the news and you are out there and I am watching the Olympics and seeing all those sporting things. It certainly does come back into my mind.'

He asked what the future held for me now I'd retired from professional sport and I explained that I was looking forward to getting married again, having a family and concentrating on my business. 'I haven't decided what I want to do in life,' Tom said, somewhat wistfully. 'I don't know if I ever will. I have been doing what I am doing at the moment because I really enjoy it. I was married, then divorced, and I have a teenage daughter who lives in another state and [spends time with me] on school holidays. What am I going to do for the next twenty years? I'm kind of hoping that my daughter would like to travel and we could do a bit of exploring together but that's a few years off. '

Then Tom paused and asked a question that had obviously been on his mind. 'How did you find my number?' 'It wasn't easy,' I said. 'What path did you follow?' he asked, not to be put off. 'There are some constants in my life but only a few people that were around at that stage that are still around.' I told him the search had started with the electoral roll. 'Didn't do you any good, did it?' he laughed. 'I got off the electoral roll many years ago. It was actually when I was driving trucks. I was moving furniture and I was given a job on a Saturday and there was an election. So I didn't get time to go and vote at all that day because I was unloading a truck and they fined me. I didn't register to vote again. How did you find me?' I told him it was through Facebook. 'Uh, it's amazing how you find people,' he quipped, shaking his head. 'I thought you might have found me through my supervisor at the time, who is still in my life. He's actually married to my ex-wife.' 'Really?' I said, surprised at this bit of personal information. I wondered how he felt about that and how that personal situation had unfolded for them all. The more we talked, the more detailed a picture I was building of his life.

Tom told me he lived close to the scene of the accident for a short period several years afterwards. 'How was that?' I asked, curious as to whether it had jogged his memory or given him any nightmares. 'I was driving past it every single day for six months,' he said. 'I never thought, "I don't want to be here." Maybe that was because I was forced to get back in the truck and get on with my life. They drove me straight from the police station back to the truck. It was a bad accident but driving past there wasn't something that brought back memories.'

I asked how he'd felt when he saw me in the hotel lobby— especially when he saw me in the wheelchair. 'I was certainly nervous,' he said. 'I did ring my boss this morning and say, "By the way, I'm out for a few hours this afternoon and this is what I am going to do." Not only is he my boss, he is almost a brother. I've worked with him now for eleven years. He is one of the few people that know. Not a lot of people do. It's not something that you run around and tell everyone.' 'What did he say,' I asked, interested in his response. 'He said, "Okay, no worries. Give me a call this afternoon and let me know how it goes." What did I think I was going to get out of today? I don't know. Maybe it has brought a bit of closure for me as well knowing that you've certainly been around and achieved things and been able to have a good life albeit a different life from mine. Maybe it helped me close that chapter.'

I felt for him then. I wondered if he had blocked out the accident so that the memory of it had sat in the back of his mind all these years, waiting for the right trigger to bring it back into his consciousness. 'It's been a great thing,' I said, referring to our meeting. 'Today I met you and we're not that dissimilar in terms of knowing what is right and wrong and I think it was a big thing for you to come here and I'm glad you did. I hope it allows you to put it away and the same goes for me. You're a nice guy. You were advised to do what you did at the time and you were younger than me. I have a sense of closure around that day now that you have clarified what happened at least as far as you are concerned—and I thank you for that. We can go on and if I see you down the street in years to come I can say "G'day" rather than never knowing who you were.'

> ... belief in yourself, commitment to your family, responsibility in your business or work, and giving back to your community. Together, they harmonise to provide the balance that helps sustain us in the good times and the bad.

Tom smiled and I felt his relief, as if it were washing over me too. It seemed the perfect note on which to end. He stood up and we shook hands. I think it's unlikely we will ever meet again—but who knows? Stranger things have happened in my life. In forgiving the truck driver I felt as if a dead weight had been lifted from my shoulders. When Tom walked out of the room and closed the door behind him, I stood up, which I can do for very short periods of time, resting on my left leg. I stretched my back and neck and arms and the first thought that came into my mind about the meeting was how sorry I felt for him. I drew no comfort from the fact that life had obviously dealt him some poor cards, too. I had confronted my fear about meeting him. Now I knew what had happened that day. Never again would I have to come up with scenarios to fill in the gaps. It was an accident, and the man who was driving the truck was sorry— and I could live with that.

It dawned on me why the meeting was so powerful—what you hold onto in life holds onto you. That's what I learnt that day. I had faced my fear. It was not enough to talk about what had happened, I had to have this meeting—I had to go through the process—to get it right in my own mind and be free of it. I no longer felt the need to hold on. I felt a sense of closure.

A FUTURE BRIGHT WITH PROMISE

Preceded by a tartan-kilted piper playing 'Amazing Grace', Amanda walked down the path towards me on our wedding day. She looked breathtakingly beautiful in her ankle-length, gold-sequinned dress and I couldn't quite believe my good fortune—that this wonderful woman was about to become my wife. There wasn't a dry eye in the crowd as a solo vocalist followed with the Maori love song 'Pokarekare Ana', referencing Amanda's New Zealand background. Many of our friends and family knew the words and sang along, creating a soulful sound that seemed to catch the light afternoon breeze and float gently around us.

I looked at Amanda and was filled with overwhelming love. At that moment I knew I had my gold medal. It wasn't a shiny piece of metal hanging off an Olympic ribbon, but a future bright with the promise of love and good times. It had taken forty-two years but I was finally at the point where all the pieces of my life had come together.

We had written our own vows, and exchanged them by the water outside the Italian restaurant where we'd chosen to hold our wedding reception. After the ceremony, we moved inside to celebrate with family and dear friends. With a five-piece jazz band in the background, my dad sang 'For Once in My Life' and almost brought the house down. The speeches were uplifting. John Young and David Knight both stood up and spoke, as did Amanda's brother Calvin, then Amanda herself, and last of all me. At the end Amanda and I took to the dance floor for our first spin as husband and wife to Eva Cassidy's verson of 'At Last (My Love Has Come Along)'. It was perfect.

Later, as Amanda and I toasted absent loved ones, I thought of my half-brother Kenny, who died suddenly in November. Although I hadn't seen him very often, his death nonetheless came as a shock, a reminder that no one knows what the future holds. A lot of people take living for granted, all the time fearing death. But I don't. If I were to die tomorrow I'd have no regrets. I've been lucky. I was given a second chance after the accident, when it would have been so easy to let go, and not only have I turned my life around and played my best hand with the cards I was dealt, I've learnt a few lessons along the way.

I believe there are four keys to a successful life—belief in yourself, commitment to your family, responsibility in your business or work, and giving back to your community. Together, they harmonise to provide the balance that helps sustain us in the good times and the bad.

I don't need to be told that things don't always work out the way you want. Nothing has ever come easily to me. I'm not one of those people who glide effortlessly through life achieving their goals on the first attempt. That's not my story. It didn't happen that way in Hawaii or in the middle of the English

Channel or at the Sydney Olympics or the Beijing Paralympics or even in my first marriage. I've had to work at getting things right. I believe that message resonates strongly with people. Life can be difficult and challenging. We all need to *believe* that whatever happens, whatever we face, dreams really *can* come true.

Maurie told me there are only two true emotions in life— love and fear. Fear is not something I hold onto. When Maurie made me realise I was running away from the emotional grief caused by my mother's death so long ago, I tried to face it as honestly as I could, just as I did the truck driver whose mistake cost me the use of my legs. Forgiveness is a powerful act. People ask me now how meeting him affected me. What purpose did it serve? I believe it allowed me to truly look at what I've learnt over the past twenty years.

I am embarking on a new chapter in my life. After Beijing I announced my retirement from professional sport. While that doesn't mean I won't be involved in sporting events, particularly those that raise money for the foundation and kids in wheelchairs, it does mean the focus of my energy has shifted to my business and my new life.

Meeting the truck driver helped me make this transition. It untied me from the event that caused my paraplegia and in turn allowed me to shed the skin of a professional sportsman and look forward to a different life with endless possibilities. I have come full circle.